Adrenal Adventures

Exploring the Physiology and Function of the Adrenal Glands

Brandon Rivers

Table of Contents

1 Introduction to the Adrenals

Nestled atop each kidney, the adrenal glands are small but mighty endocrine organs, vital for life. Their yellowish-brown hue belies the complex biochemical processes occurring within, shaping our response to stress and regulating essential bodily functions. These paired glands, each about the size of a walnut, are truly remarkable examples of sophisticated biological engineering. Understanding their intricate anatomy forms the foundation for comprehending their multifaceted roles.

The adrenal cortex, the outer layer, is responsible for the production of steroid hormones. These include glucocorticoids like cortisol, essential for regulating metabolism, the immune system, and blood sugar levels; mineralocorticoids, such as aldosterone, which play a crucial role in maintaining sodium and potassium balance and consequently, blood pressure; and androgens, contributing to secondary sexual characteristics. The different zones within the cortex—the zona glomerulosa, fasciculata, and reticularis—each specialize in synthesizing distinct steroid hormones. Each zone's cellular structure and enzyme complement contributes to the precise regulation of the steroidogenic pathways.

In contrast, the adrenal medulla, the inner core, functions as part of the sympathetic nervous system. It primarily synthesizes and releases catecholamines—epinephrine (adrenaline) and norepinephrine (noradrenaline)—potent hormones crucial for the "fight-or-flight" response. This rapid response system prepares the body for stressful situations, increasing heart rate, blood pressure, and alertness. Understanding the interplay between the cortex and medulla reveals the comprehensive role of these glands in maintaining homeostasis.

Our understanding of the adrenals hasn't always been as complete. Early anatomical studies provided only a rudimentary insight into their function. It wasn't until the 19th and 20th centuries that researchers began to unravel the specific roles of adrenal hormones. Early experiments, often involving adrenalectomy in animals, revealed the critical nature of these glands for survival. The discovery of specific hormones, their synthesis pathways, and their precise physiological effects constituted pivotal advancements in the field. Thomas Addison's description of Addison's disease in 1855, marked a crucial turning point—the first clear recognition of adrenal insufficiency and its life-threatening consequences. This led to further investigations into adrenal function and pathology, accelerating our understanding of these vital organs and shaping modern endocrinology. Subsequent research, employing techniques like chromatography and radioimmunoassays, allowed scientists to precisely measure hormone levels, deepening our understanding of their regulation and the consequences of their imbalance. The development of sophisticated imaging techniques, including CT and MRI scans, further enhanced our diagnostic capabilities, enabling clinicians to visualize adrenal glands and identify pathologies with unprecedented accuracy. This continuous evolution of research methods underscores the ongoing importance of studying adrenal function and its implications for human health.

The study of the adrenal glands presents an engaging intersection of anatomy, physiology, biochemistry, and pathology. The complexity of their internal organization, the intricate interplay of various hormonal pathways, and the significant implications of their dysfunction make them a captivating subject for medical and scientific exploration. The ongoing development of novel diagnostic and therapeutic strategies ensures the continued relevance and importance of comprehensive knowledge about these small but crucial endocrine glands. Therefore, a thorough understanding of adrenal function and the clinical implications of its disruption lays the groundwork for a deeper appreciation of human physiology and effective patient care.

1.1 Adrenal Anatomy

Nestled atop each kidney, like tiny pyramids, lie the adrenal glands. These small, vital organs, though seemingly insignificant in size, orchestrate a complex symphony of hormonal responses crucial for life itself. Their location, snugly encased within the protective embrace of the retroperitoneal space, underscores their importance – shielded yet readily accessible to the bloodstream. Imagine them as silent conductors, directing a crucial orchestra of biochemical processes.

Each adrenal gland, itself a fascinating miniature ecosystem, is divided into two distinct functional zones: the cortex and the medulla. The outer cortex, the larger of the two, is further subdivided into three layers – the zona glomerulosa, the zona fasciculata, and the zona reticularis – each responsible for the production of specific steroid hormones. Think of it as a layered cake, each layer offering a unique and essential ingredient to our overall hormonal balance. This intricate layering isn't merely aesthetic; it reflects the distinct biochemical pathways involved in hormone synthesis.

The zona glomerulosa, the outermost layer, specializes in the production of mineralocorticoids, predominantly aldosterone. Aldosterone, a critical regulator of electrolyte balance, acts primarily on the kidneys to control sodium and potassium levels, influencing blood volume and pressure. This process is vital for maintaining homeostasis, ensuring the proper balance of fluids within the body. A disruption in this delicate balance can have significant consequences.

Moving deeper into the adrenal cortex, we encounter the zona fasciculata. This expansive middle layer is the primary site of glucocorticoid production, particularly cortisol. Cortisol is arguably the most versatile hormone produced by the adrenals, deeply influencing metabolism, stress response, and the immune system. Its actions are wide-ranging, impacting everything from blood sugar regulation to the body's reaction to infection and inflammation. Understanding cortisol's multifaceted role is key to grasping the full significance of adrenal function.

Finally, the innermost layer of the adrenal cortex, the zona reticularis, contributes to the production of adrenal androgens, steroid hormones that influence sexual characteristics and contribute to overall metabolic processes. Although produced in smaller quantities compared to cortisol or aldosterone, these androgens play a subtle yet significant role in the complex hormonal interplay within the body, especially during development and throughout life. Their subtle influence helps illustrate the intricate nature of adrenal function.

In stark contrast to the steroid-producing cortex, the

adrenal medulla, the inner core of the gland, acts as a rapid-response system, primarily secreting catecholamines, namely epinephrine and norepinephrine. These hormones, also known as adrenaline and noradrenaline, respectively, are intimately involved in the body's fight-or-flight response, mobilizing resources during stressful situations. They surge into the bloodstream, rapidly altering heart rate, blood pressure, and metabolic processes, preparing the body for immediate action.

The intricate vascular network surrounding the adrenal glands further highlights their strategic importance. A rich supply of blood vessels ensures efficient delivery of hormones into the circulation, allowing for rapid response to changing physiological demands. This highly efficient delivery system underlines the speed at which the adrenal glands can react and adapt to the body's needs. Think of it as a highly efficient distribution network, ensuring that vital hormones reach their destinations swiftly and effectively.

The precise anatomical location, the distinct layering of the cortex, the rapid-response capabilities of the medulla—all these features contribute to the adrenal glands' pivotal role in maintaining homeostasis. Understanding the adrenal anatomy is not merely an academic exercise; it's the cornerstone to comprehending the complex interplay of hormones that govern our daily lives and our responses to stress and disease. The intricacies of the adrenal glands emphasize the elegant precision of the human body and its remarkable ability to adapt and maintain balance. It is a testament to the sophistication of biological systems. Failing to appreciate this complexity would be a serious oversight in any study of endocrinology or physiology. Their significance goes far beyond their diminutive size.

1.2 Adrenal History

Early observations of the adrenal glands, those small, vital organs perched atop our kidneys, were largely anatomical. Ancient civilizations, from Egyptians to Greeks, noted their presence, but their function remained shrouded in mystery. Think of the painstaking dissections performed centuries ago, revealing only the glands' physical attributes – their shape, their location, their proximity to the kidneys. The true significance, however, lay dormant. The scientific understanding of the adrenals began to blossom in the 19th century, spurred by advancements in physiological research. Thomas Addison's detailed description of a debilitating disease, now bearing his name, proved pivotal. Addison's disease, characterized by adrenal insufficiency, linked specific clinical features—fatigue, weight loss, low blood pressure—to the dysfunction of these previously enigmatic glands. This landmark observation shifted the focus from mere anatomy to the critical role of the adrenal glands in maintaining overall bodily health.

Further progress demanded a deeper delve into the biochemistry of the adrenal glands. The isolation and identification of hormones produced by these organs—cortisol, aldosterone, epinephrine, and norepinephrine—represented monumental steps forward in the early to mid-20th century. The detailed chemical characterization of these hormones illuminated their distinct actions and opened avenues for research into their specific functions. The development of sophisticated techniques, including chromatography and spectroscopy, allowed researchers to isolate and identify these critical molecules, proving that the adrenals were more than just anatomical curiosities; they were endocrine powerhouses.

Understanding the mechanisms of hormone production within the adrenals became crucial. Researchers discovered that the different zones within the adrenal cortex—the zona glomerulosa, fasciculata, and reticularis—produced distinct hormones, each with specific regulatory pathways and target organs. This refined our understanding, moving beyond a simple description of the adrenals as a whole to a more complex picture involving compartmentalized hormone synthesis. The elegant interplay of enzymes, feedback loops, and regulatory signals within these zones became a central focus, leading to a deeper understanding of adrenal physiology.

Moreover, the discovery of the renin-angiotensin-aldosterone system (RAAS) shed light on the intricate regulation of blood pressure and fluid balance. This cascade of events, beginning with the kidney and culminating in aldosterone release from the adrenal glands, illustrated the interconnectedness of different organ systems and the central role of the adrenals in maintaining homeostasis. It was a significant turning point, demonstrating that the adrenals weren't isolated actors but rather integrated players within a complex, finely tuned physiological orchestra.

The development of sophisticated analytical techniques, such as radioimmunoassays, revolutionized the ability to measure hormone levels precisely. This made possible the accurate diagnosis of adrenal disorders and allowed for monitoring the efficacy of therapeutic interventions. Before these precise methods, diagnosing adrenal issues relied heavily on the presentation of clinical symptoms. The ability to quantitatively assess hormone levels provided an objective measure of adrenal function.

The 20th century also saw significant advancements in our understanding of the stress response and the role of the adrenal medulla. The work of Hans Selye on stress, and the identification of the fight-or-flight response, highlighted the importance of epinephrine and norepinephrine in the body's response to threat. This understanding linked the adrenals not only to homeostatic regulation but also to crucial survival mechanisms. These insights linked adrenal function to the body's adaptive responses to a wide range of stimuli.

In the late 20th and early 21st centuries, the use of advanced imaging techniques, such as computed tomography (CT) and magnetic resonance imaging (MRI), allowed for precise visualization of adrenal gland anatomy. These techniques enabled the detection of tumors and other abnormalities, improving both the diagnosis and management of adrenal disorders. The ability to directly visualize the adrenal glands revolutionized diagnostic capabilities and dramatically changed clinical approaches to various adrenal-related pathologies. This marked a pivotal shift from relying solely on indirect measurements to a direct assessment of the gland's structural integrity. It further cemented the importance of the adrenal glands in health and disease.

The history of adrenal gland research is a testament to the power of persistent inquiry and the interconnectedness of scientific disciplines. From initial anatomical observations to the precise molecular understanding of hormone synthesis and regulation, our journey has been marked by significant discoveries that continue to shape our approach to endocrine disorders. The ongoing research on the adrenal glands promises even more profound insights into their complex functions and their implications for human health. The ongoing research remains an exciting endeavor.

2 Cortisol's Crucial Role

The intricate dance of cortisol synthesis begins within the adrenal cortex, a fascinating anatomical region. Here, cholesterol undergoes a series of enzymatic transformations, a carefully orchestrated cascade involving 21-hydroxylase, 17-alpha-hydroxylase, and 11-beta-hydroxylase, crucial enzymes that convert cholesterol to pregnenolone, then to 17-hydroxypregnenolone, and finally culminating in cortisol. This finely tuned process ensures a constant, yet adaptable, supply of this vital hormone. Disruptions at any stage can have significant consequences, leading to hormonal imbalances and associated pathologies. Understanding these intricate biochemical pathways is fundamental to comprehending cortisol's multifaceted roles in the body.

Cortisol's release is a masterclass in endocrine regulation. The hypothalamic-pituitary-adrenal (HPA) axis acts as the conductor of this complex symphony. The hypothalamus, the brain's command center, releases corticotropin-releasing hormone (CRH) in response to various stimuli, including stress, circadian rhythm, and hypoglycemia. This triggers the anterior pituitary gland to secrete adrenocorticotropic hormone (ACTH), which then travels through the bloodstream to the adrenal glands, stimulating the production and release of cortisol. This feedback loop ensures that cortisol levels remain within a tightly controlled range, adapting to the body's fluctuating needs. Negative feedback mechanisms, primarily mediated by cortisol itself, prevent overproduction.

Cortisol exerts far-reaching effects throughout the body. Its influence on metabolism is particularly profound. Cortisol promotes gluconeogenesis, the production of glucose from non-carbohydrate sources, providing a readily available energy source during periods of stress or fasting. It also increases protein breakdown in muscle tissue and enhances lipolysis, the breakdown of fats. While these processes are essential for survival in challenging situations, prolonged exposure to elevated cortisol levels can lead to detrimental effects, including muscle wasting, increased abdominal fat, and impaired glucose tolerance. These effects highlight the crucial balance required for optimal metabolic health.

Beyond its metabolic influence, cortisol plays a central role in the immune system. It acts as a powerful anti-inflammatory and immunosuppressant agent. This property is essential in controlling inflammation and preventing overactive immune responses. However, chronic elevation of cortisol can suppress the immune system, making the individual more susceptible to infections and impairing wound healing. This duality illustrates the necessity for appropriately regulated cortisol levels for maintaining a robust and effectively functioning immune response.

The role of cortisol in the stress response is paramount, affecting both physical and psychological well-being. When faced with stressors, the HPA axis is activated, leading to a surge in cortisol secretion, preparing the body for "fight or flight." This acute response is adaptive, enhancing alertness, increasing heart rate, and diverting resources to essential functions. However, chronic stress, which leads to sustained elevated cortisol levels, disrupts the delicate balance, resulting in a cascade of negative consequences, ranging from impaired cognitive function and mood disturbances to increased risk of cardiovascular disease and other chronic illnesses. Understanding this crucial role of cortisol in stress management is essential in developing strategies for coping with stress and promoting overall well-being.

In conclusion, cortisol is far more than just a hormone. It's a master regulator, involved in a multitude of critical physiological processes, affecting everything from our metabolic rate and immune response to our ability to manage stress. A comprehensive understanding of cortisol's synthesis, regulation, and diverse effects is essential for appreciating its fundamental role in maintaining health and well-being. Its crucial role underscores the importance of maintaining hormonal balance and the implications of prolonged exposure to elevated cortisol levels. Further exploration into cortisol's interaction with other hormones and systems will provide deeper insights into this remarkable molecule and its intricate contribution to overall health. This complex interplay necessitates a nuanced approach in understanding its influence on human physiology. The intricate details of cortisol's impact are far-reaching and highlight the body's remarkable adaptive capabilities, but also its vulnerability when this finely tuned system is disrupted.

2.1 Cortisol Synthesis

The synthesis of cortisol, a steroid hormone crucial for life, begins in the adrenal cortex, specifically within the zona fasciculata. This process, a complex interplay of enzymatic reactions, is meticulously regulated to maintain homeostasis. It all starts with cholesterol, the fundamental building block. Cholesterol, obtained from LDLs in the bloodstream or synthesized de novo within the adrenal cells, undergoes a series of transformations.

The first major step involves the conversion of cholesterol to pregnenolone, catalyzed by the enzyme cholesterol desmolase (CYP11A1). This enzyme, located in the mitochondria, is the rate-limiting step in the entire pathway, meaning its activity directly controls the overall production of cortisol. Factors like ACTH (adrenocorticotropic hormone) from the anterior pituitary gland significantly influence cholesterol desmolase activity, ensuring the body produces the appropriate amount of cortisol to meet demands. Think of it as a master switch, carefully regulating the flow of the entire process.

Pregnenolone, now formed, embarks on a series of transformations, moving between the mitochondria and the endoplasmic reticulum. It's a fascinating journey, a dance between cellular compartments. Each step is facilitated by a specific enzyme. First, pregnenolone is converted to 17-hydroxypregnenolone by 17-hydroxylase (CYP17A1). Then, another enzyme, 21-hydroxylase (CYP21A2), takes over and converts 17-hydroxypregnenolone to 11-deoxycortisol. Deficiencies in any of these crucial enzymes can lead to serious hormonal imbalances and conditions. This is why understanding each step is absolutely vital.

The final step, the conversion of 11-deoxycortisol to cortisol, occurs in the mitochondria via 11-hydroxylase (CYP11B1). This enzyme completes the synthesis, resulting in the secretion of cortisol into the bloodstream. Cortisol then binds to its receptors within target cells, triggering a cascade of biological effects. This includes regulating blood glucose levels, suppressing the inflammatory response, and influencing mood and cognitive function. This delicate balance highlights the importance of maintaining proper cortisol synthesis.

The entire process, from cholesterol to cortisol, is highly regulated, not only by ACTH but also by other factors such as glucocorticoid receptor feedback and availability of the necessary enzymes and substrates. These intricate control mechanisms prevent both cortisol deficiency and excess, conditions that can have profound implications on health. It's a precise, finely tuned system that constantly adapts to changing physiological demands, ensuring the body's overall well-being. Understanding this detailed mechanism reveals the inherent complexity of endocrine regulation, crucial for appreciating the significance of cortisol in maintaining a healthy balance.

Dysregulation in any part of this synthetic pathway can have far-reaching consequences. For example, a deficiency in 21-hydroxylase, a common cause of congenital adrenal hyperplasia, disrupts cortisol synthesis, leading to an accumulation of cortisol precursors and excessive androgen production. This can cause virilization in females and precocious puberty in males. Understanding the specific enzyme deficiencies enables clinicians to accurately diagnose and treat these conditions effectively. The clinical implications are far-reaching, and a comprehensive understanding of this synthesis process is crucial to effective diagnosis and patient care.

Moreover, environmental factors and lifestyle choices can also indirectly influence cortisol synthesis. Stress, sleep deprivation, and poor diet can affect the hypothalamic-pituitary-adrenal (HPA) axis, altering ACTH secretion and consequently cortisol production. Chronic stress, in particular, can lead to prolonged elevation of cortisol levels, potentially damaging the body's systems over time. These facts emphasize the importance of adopting a holistic approach to maintain healthy cortisol levels, encompassing both internal hormonal balance and external lifestyle choices.

In summary, cortisol synthesis is a remarkably intricate process, involving multiple enzymes and intracellular compartments. It's a finely-tuned dance orchestrated by hormones and feedback mechanisms, all working together to maintain the delicate balance of the body's physiology. Each step is essential, and any disruption can lead to significant health consequences. Understanding this fundamental process is not merely academic; it's critical for comprehending the body's response to stress, inflammation, and overall metabolic health. It allows for a deeper appreciation of endocrine function and provides insight into the clinical management of hormonal disorders. The knowledge gained here lays the groundwork for subsequent chapters exploring cortisol regulation, effects, and relevant clinical implications.

2.2 Cortisol Regulation

The hypothalamus, that tiny but mighty region of your brain, acts as the primary conductor of the cortisol orchestra. It senses stress – whether it's the looming deadline, a difficult conversation, or even just a demanding workout – and responds by releasing corticotropin-releasing hormone (CRH). This CRH then travels to the anterior pituitary gland, stimulating the release of adrenocorticotropic hormone (ACTH). Think of ACTH as the baton, carrying the signal onward.

ACTH's journey leads it to the adrenal glands, specifically the adrenal cortex, where it binds to receptors on the cells responsible for cortisol production. This binding initiates a cascade of enzymatic reactions, ultimately leading to the synthesis and release of cortisol into the bloodstream. It's a beautifully orchestrated process, a testament to the intricate communication network within our bodies. The precise control of this multi-step process is essential; too little cortisol, and we risk adrenal insufficiency, while excessive cortisol production can lead to Cushing's syndrome. Both conditions highlight the vital importance of maintaining a delicate balance.

Feedback mechanisms are crucial to ensure that cortisol levels remain within the optimal range. Once cortisol reaches sufficient levels in the bloodstream, it exerts a negative feedback effect on both the hypothalamus and the pituitary gland. This feedback loop is a sophisticated self-regulating system. It prevents overproduction of CRH and ACTH, thus preventing excessive cortisol release. This intricate regulatory process is akin to a thermostat controlling room temperature; it constantly monitors levels and adjusts output accordingly, ensuring a stable internal environment. Disruptions in this feedback system are often at the heart of many adrenal disorders.

Maintaining a healthy lifestyle is vital for supporting healthy cortisol regulation. Chronic stress, poor sleep, and an unhealthy diet can significantly impact this delicate balance. Regular exercise, a balanced diet rich in nutrients, and sufficient sleep contribute to optimal adrenal function. These lifestyle choices help minimize the body's need to constantly produce cortisol in response to sustained stress. Incorporating stress-reduction techniques like meditation or yoga can further improve this balance. We are not passive recipients of stress; we have the power to shape our responses and mitigate the long-term consequences of chronic stress on our adrenal system.

Beyond lifestyle choices, understanding your individual stress triggers is crucial. Identifying and managing these triggers actively contributes to the maintenance of a balanced cortisol level. This involves developing coping mechanisms to address stressors effectively. This might include setting realistic goals, practicing assertiveness, learning to say "no," or finding healthy ways to release tension. This personal insight is transformative; it empowers individuals to address the root cause of their stress, rather than simply treating the symptoms. The goal isn't to eliminate all stress—that's unrealistic and arguably unhealthy—but rather to manage stress effectively, preventing it from overwhelming the adrenal system.

Furthermore, seeking professional help is a sign of strength, not weakness. A healthcare provider can provide personalized advice based on your individual circumstances and help diagnose and treat any underlying adrenal disorders. This might involve blood tests to measure cortisol levels and other relevant hormones. Further testing could include imaging techniques to evaluate the structure and function of the adrenal glands. Early detection and intervention are crucial in preventing severe health consequences associated with both cortisol deficiency and excess. Ignoring potential problems can lead to complications, while early intervention often leads to improved health outcomes.

In conclusion, the regulation of cortisol is a complex and finely tuned process, essential for maintaining overall health and well-being. It involves a sophisticated interplay between the hypothalamus, pituitary gland, and adrenal cortex. While the body possesses robust self-regulating mechanisms, our lifestyle choices and stress management strategies profoundly impact this process. By prioritizing healthy habits, managing stress effectively, and seeking professional help when needed, we can support optimal cortisol regulation and contribute to our overall well-being. Remember, understanding your body is the first step towards a healthier, happier you. This knowledge empowers you to make informed decisions that benefit your long-term health. This process of self-awareness is a continuous journey, not a destination.

2.3 Cortisol Effects

Cortisol, the primary glucocorticoid hormone produced by the adrenal cortex, exerts profound and wide-ranging effects throughout the body. Its influence extends far beyond simply mediating the stress response; it plays a crucial role in regulating metabolism, immune function, and even cardiovascular health. Understanding these effects is paramount for appreciating the adrenal gland's overall significance in maintaining homeostasis.

Its impact on metabolism is multifaceted and significant. Cortisol promotes gluconeogenesis, the process of creating glucose from non-carbohydrate sources like amino acids and glycerol. This is particularly important during periods of fasting or stress, when glucose supplies are low. Conversely, cortisol inhibits glucose uptake in peripheral tissues, ensuring that glucose remains available for the brain and other vital organs. This intricate balancing act is crucial for maintaining blood glucose levels within a narrow physiological range. In addition, cortisol influences lipid metabolism, promoting lipolysis (breakdown of fats) in some tissues while simultaneously stimulating lipogenesis (fat synthesis) in others, a complex interplay vital for energy storage and utilization. Finally, cortisol affects protein metabolism, promoting protein catabolism (breakdown) in muscle tissue to provide amino acids for gluconeogenesis.

The immune system is profoundly influenced by cortisol. It acts as a potent immunosuppressant, reducing inflammation and suppressing immune cell activity. While this is beneficial in mitigating harmful inflammatory responses during injury or infection, chronic elevation of cortisol can leave the body vulnerable to infections and impair the body's ability to fight off diseases. This immunosuppressive effect occurs through the inhibition of various immune cells, including lymphocytes (T cells and B cells) and macrophages. The precise mechanisms by which cortisol achieves this inhibition are complex and involve interactions with multiple intracellular signaling pathways. A well-balanced cortisol level is essential for optimal immune function, avoiding both over\item and under-active states.

Cortisol's influence extends to cardiovascular function, impacting blood pressure and vascular tone. While acute cortisol release can contribute to increased blood pressure during the stress response, chronic elevation can lead to negative cardiovascular consequences. Prolonged exposure to high cortisol levels can result in increased vascular resistance, contributing to hypertension and an increased risk of cardiovascular disease. It's important to remember this is not a simple relationship; rather, cortisol interacts with other hormones and signaling pathways to produce its effects on the cardiovascular system.

Beyond these major effects, cortisol influences numerous other physiological processes. It plays a role in fluid balance through its interactions with the kidneys. It's involved in bone metabolism and calcium regulation, potentially affecting bone density. Moreover, cortisol has been implicated in cognitive function, mood regulation, and sleep-wake cycles. A delicate balance is essential; insufficient cortisol can lead to fatigue, weakness, and cognitive impairment, while excessive levels can be associated with anxiety, mood disorders, and sleep disturbances. Proper adrenal function and carefully regulated cortisol secretion are therefore key to maintaining overall well-being.

Maintaining healthy cortisol levels is crucial for optimal health. While acute stress and its resultant cortisol surge are normal physiological responses, chronic stress and prolonged cortisol elevation can have detrimental effects. Lifestyle choices play a significant role in mitigating chronic stress. Prioritizing sufficient sleep, engaging in regular physical activity, and adopting stress-reducing techniques such as meditation or yoga can help to regulate cortisol levels. A balanced diet, rich in fruits, vegetables, and whole grains, can also contribute to overall well-being and hormonal balance. A holistic approach, combining lifestyle adjustments with appropriate medical attention when necessary, is essential in maintaining optimal cortisol levels and supporting overall health. Ultimately, understanding cortisol's diverse effects enables us to adopt a more informed approach to promoting both physical and mental health. Recognizing the critical role cortisol plays in various physiological processes empowers individuals to make lifestyle choices and seek medical advice when needed to ensure a healthy balance.

3 Aldosterone: Sodium's Guardian

The adrenal cortex, a vital part of our endocrine system, produces aldosterone, a steroid hormone crucial for maintaining our body's sodium balance. This seemingly simple task is actually incredibly complex, involving intricate feedback loops and precise hormonal interactions. Think of aldosterone as the diligent guardian of sodium, ensuring its levels remain within a narrow, carefully regulated range. Without this tight control, serious complications such as dehydration, dangerously low blood pressure, and even cardiac arrest could result.

Aldosterone's production begins with the stimulation of the adrenal cortex cells by angiotensin II, a powerful peptide hormone part of the renin-angiotensin-aldosterone system (RAAS). This system is activated in response to low blood volume or low blood pressure, triggering a cascade of events that ultimately lead to aldosterone secretion. Another pivotal player in this process is potassium. High levels of potassium in the blood directly stimulate the adrenal cortex to release more aldosterone. The complex interplay of angiotensin II and potassium concentration serves as a finely tuned mechanism to ensure appropriate aldosterone production. This finely tuned process ensures that aldosterone secretion directly addresses the body's needs.

Once released into the bloodstream, aldosterone travels to its primary target organs: the kidneys. There, it binds to specific receptors located in the cells of the distal tubules and collecting ducts. This binding initiates a series of intracellular events leading to the increased reabsorption of sodium from the urine back into the bloodstream. Simultaneously, potassium is secreted into the urine. This exchange, orchestrated by aldosterone, is critical for maintaining electrolyte balance. It's a carefully balanced act, and disturbances here have far-reaching consequences.

The effects of aldosterone extend beyond simple sodium and potassium regulation. By increasing sodium reabsorption, aldosterone also causes water reabsorption. This is because water follows sodium due to osmotic pressure. This increased water retention leads to an expansion of blood volume and increased blood pressure. This helps restore blood pressure to normal when it's dangerously low. This is why aldosterone is so critical during periods of dehydration or blood loss. Its effect on blood pressure is a crucial mechanism of maintaining cardiovascular health.

Conversely, aldosterone deficiency, as seen in Addison's disease, results in decreased sodium reabsorption, leading to hyponatremia (low blood sodium), hypovolemia (low blood volume), and hypotension (low blood pressure). These consequences highlight the essential role of aldosterone in maintaining fluid and electrolyte balance. The body's inability to effectively regulate sodium results in a cascade of negative effects, including dangerously low blood pressure. These patients often require regular medication to replace their deficient aldosterone.

Conversely, excess aldosterone, as seen in primary aldosteronism (Conn's syndrome), can cause hypernatremia (high blood sodium), hypokalemia (low blood potassium), and hypertension (high blood pressure). The imbalance caused by excessive aldosterone can severely impact cardiovascular health. Individuals with primary aldosteronism often experience symptoms like muscle weakness, increased thirst and urination, and elevated blood pressure. Management frequently involves medication to inhibit aldosterone production or carefully regulated dietary modifications.

Understanding aldosterone's intricate role in maintaining sodium balance is crucial for comprehending several physiological processes, from blood pressure regulation to electrolyte homeostasis. The complex interplay of hormones and feedback mechanisms involved in aldosterone production and action illustrates the exquisite precision of our endocrine system. Proper functioning of the RAAS and the responsiveness of the kidneys are integral to preserving this balance. Disruptions to this delicate equilibrium can have far-reaching and potentially life-threatening consequences. Recognizing the importance of aldosterone's role, therefore, is paramount to understanding overall endocrine health. This knowledge facilitates accurate diagnosis and appropriate treatment for a multitude of conditions, underscoring the significance of this often-overlooked hormone in maintaining overall health.

3.1 Aldosterone Production

The adrenal cortex, specifically the zona glomerulosa, is the birthplace of aldosterone. Its production, a finely tuned process, hinges on a complex interplay of hormonal signals and enzymatic reactions. The renin-angiotensin-aldosterone system (RAAS) plays a central role; a decrease in blood pressure or sodium levels triggers renin release from the juxtaglomerular cells in the kidneys. Renin, in turn, initiates a cascade, converting angiotensinogen to angiotensin I, then angiotensin II, a potent vasoconstrictor and stimulator of aldosterone secretion. Angiotensin II directly acts on the zona glomerulosa cells, stimulating aldosterone synthesis and release.

This isn't the entire picture, though. Potassium levels also exert significant influence. Elevated potassium directly stimulates aldosterone production, acting independently of the RAAS pathway. This is a crucial feedback mechanism, ensuring potassium homeostasis is maintained. High potassium levels are directly sensed by the zona glomerulosa cells, prompting increased aldosterone synthesis; the hormone then promotes potassium excretion in the kidneys, thereby lowering blood potassium.

Corticotropin-releasing hormone (CRH) and adrenocorticotropic hormone (ACTH), primarily associated with cortisol regulation, also subtly affect aldosterone. While their impact is less pronounced than that of angiotensin II or potassium, chronic exposure to elevated ACTH can stimulate aldosterone production. This complex interplay highlights the intricate interconnectedness of the hypothalamic-pituitary-adrenal (HPA) axis and the RAAS. Understanding this interconnectedness is essential for grasping the nuances of aldosterone regulation.

The synthesis of aldosterone itself is a multi-step biochemical process, beginning with cholesterol. A series of enzymatic reactions, involving enzymes such as cytochrome P450 enzymes, convert cholesterol to pregnenolone, then progesterone, deoxycorticosterone (DOC), and finally, aldosterone. Each step is meticulously regulated, ensuring precise control over aldosterone production. Deficiencies or dysfunctions in any of these enzymes can lead to aldosterone deficiency or excessive production, resulting in significant clinical consequences. Think of it as a carefully orchestrated production line, each step crucial for the final product.

Furthermore, understanding the regulation of aldosterone production is vital for appreciating the body's ability to maintain fluid and electrolyte balance. Aldosterone's primary function is to promote sodium reabsorption and potassium excretion in the kidneys, leading to increased water retention and blood pressure regulation. This delicate balance is critical for cardiovascular health. Imbalances in aldosterone levels can manifest in a range of clinical conditions, from hypertension to hypokalemia, highlighting the importance of a thorough understanding of its regulatory mechanisms. Therefore, a detailed study of aldosterone production is a crucial component of understanding overall adrenal gland function.

Disruptions in this intricate process can have profound physiological consequences. For instance, conditions like primary hyperaldosteronism (Conn's syndrome), characterized by autonomous aldosterone overproduction, often lead to hypertension, hypokalemia, and metabolic alkalosis. Conversely, aldosterone deficiency, often seen in Addison's disease, results in hypotension, hyperkalemia, and metabolic acidosis. These contrasting clinical pictures emphasize the importance of maintaining a precise balance of aldosterone production. Understanding the normal physiological process of aldosterone production is essential for understanding these conditions.

The precise control over aldosterone production reflects the body's intricate mechanisms for maintaining homeostasis. Any disruption in the RAAS, potassium levels, or the enzymatic pathways involved in aldosterone synthesis can lead to significant health issues. The study of aldosterone production, therefore, goes beyond basic biochemistry and physiology; it delves into the realm of clinical medicine, providing essential knowledge for diagnosing and treating a range of endocrine disorders. The intricate regulation of aldosterone emphasizes the importance of

maintaining a delicate equilibrium within the body's systems.
Therefore, appreciating the complex interplay between the RAAS, potassium levels, and the enzymatic cascade involved in aldosterone synthesis is key to understanding the body's complex regulatory systems. It highlights the importance of a holistic understanding of endocrine function, where each hormone plays a vital role in maintaining overall health and well-being. Further exploration into the specific enzymes and their regulation will provide a more complete picture of this critical process. Detailed knowledge of this process is invaluable for future advancements in medical diagnosis and treatment. This sophisticated system represents a marvel of biological engineering.

3.2 Aldosterone Action

Aldosterone, a steroid hormone produced in the zona glomerulosa of the adrenal cortex, plays a pivotal role in maintaining sodium and potassium balance within the body. Its primary action is on the distal tubules and collecting ducts of the kidneys, where it promotes sodium reabsorption and potassium excretion. This carefully regulated process is crucial for maintaining extracellular fluid volume, blood pressure, and overall electrolyte homeostasis.
The mechanism of aldosterone action begins with its binding to a specific intracellular receptor, the mineralocorticoid receptor (MR). This receptor, located in the cytoplasm of target cells, undergoes a conformational change upon aldosterone binding, translocating to the nucleus. Once in the nucleus, the hormone-receptor complex interacts with specific DNA sequences, known as hormone response elements (HREs), initiating transcription of specific genes.

These genes encode proteins essential for sodium transport across the renal tubular epithelium.

One crucial protein upregulated by aldosterone is the epithelial sodium channel (ENaC). ENaC is a sodium channel located on the apical membrane of principal cells in the collecting duct. Aldosterone increases the expression and activity of ENaC, leading to enhanced sodium reabsorption from the tubular lumen into the cell. This sodium influx creates an electrochemical gradient, promoting potassium efflux via ROMK channels located on the apical membrane. Consequently, sodium is reabsorbed into the bloodstream, while potassium is excreted in the urine.

Furthermore, aldosterone's effects are not limited solely to ENaC regulation. It also influences the expression of the Na+/K+-ATPase, a transmembrane protein responsible for actively transporting sodium out of the cell and potassium into the cell across the basolateral membrane. By increasing Na+/K+-ATPase activity, aldosterone further enhances sodium reabsorption and contributes to the overall potassium-excretion process. This intricate interplay of channels and pumps ensures efficient sodium retention and potassium elimination, carefully balancing the body's electrolyte composition.

This tightly controlled system is under the influence of several regulatory pathways. The renin-angiotensin-aldosterone system (RAAS) plays a central role. A decrease in blood volume or blood pressure triggers the release of renin from the juxtaglomerular apparatus in the kidneys. Renin converts angiotensinogen to angiotensin I, which is subsequently converted to the potent vasoconstrictor angiotensin II by angiotensin-converting enzyme (ACE). Angiotensin II directly stimulates aldosterone secretion from the adrenal cortex, increasing sodium reabsorption and consequently blood pressure.

The potassium concentration in the blood also directly influences aldosterone release. Hyperkalemia, or elevated potassium levels, directly stimulates aldosterone production. This mechanism acts as a rapid feedback system to prevent potentially dangerous increases in extracellular potassium. Conversely, hypokalemia, or low potassium levels, suppresses aldosterone secretion. Therefore, the body meticulously regulates aldosterone production and secretion to maintain both sodium and potassium levels within a tight physiological range. This regulatory precision is essential for preserving cardiovascular health and preventing potentially life-threatening electrolyte imbalances.

Beyond its role in sodium and potassium homeostasis, aldosterone exhibits other physiological effects. For instance, it contributes to extracellular fluid volume regulation, influencing blood pressure and cardiac function. Aldosterone also interacts with other hormonal systems, impacting fluid balance and potentially influencing vascular tone and structure. While these secondary effects are less significant than its primary role in electrolyte balance, their interplay with other physiological processes highlights the complex and interconnected nature of endocrine regulation. Disruptions in aldosterone production or action can have wide-ranging effects on the body, emphasizing the significance of this vital mineralocorticoid.

Clinically, aldosterone imbalances are associated with various pathologies. Hyperaldosteronism, characterized by excessive aldosterone production, can lead to hypertension, hypokalemia, and metabolic alkalosis. Primary hyperaldosteronism, often caused by adrenal adenomas or hyperplasia, requires specific diagnostic tests and tailored management strategies. Conversely, hypoaldosteronism, or insufficient aldosterone production, can result in hyponatremia, hyperkalemia, and metabolic acidosis, conditions that often necessitate careful monitoring and hormone replacement therapy. Understanding the precise mechanisms of aldosterone action is crucial for accurate diagnosis and effective treatment of these conditions, further highlighting the pivotal role of this hormone in human health. The precise regulation of aldosterone production, its mechanisms of action at the cellular level, and its clinical significance in disease states are all areas of ongoing research, constantly expanding our comprehension of this vital hormone. Continued investigation in these critical areas promises to further refine our diagnostic and therapeutic approaches, offering improved patient care in the future.

4 Catecholamines: Fight or Flight

The adrenal medulla, nestled within the adrenal glands, is a critical player in our body's rapid response to stress. Its primary function is the synthesis and secretion of catecholamines: epinephrine (adrenaline) and norepinephrine (noradrenaline). These hormones are not merely bystanders; they are central orchestrators of the "fight-or-flight" response, a crucial survival mechanism honed over millennia. Imagine a threatening situation – your heart races, your breathing quickens, your senses sharpen. These are the hallmarks of the sympathetic nervous system's activation, triggered largely by the surge of catecholamines.

Epinephrine, the more abundant catecholamine, exerts profound effects throughout the body. It dramatically increases heart rate and contractility, boosting cardiac output and delivering oxygen-rich blood to muscles. Simultaneously, it constricts blood vessels in non-essential areas, diverting blood flow to the muscles needed for immediate action. Blood glucose levels also skyrocket, providing the muscles with readily available fuel. These changes, orchestrated by epinephrine, prepare the body for intense physical activity, be it fighting off a threat or fleeing to safety. Its effects on metabolic processes, such as glycogenolysis and lipolysis, are further examples of the rapid mobilization of energy resources. The rapid and widespread effects of epinephrine highlight its crucial role in the immediate stress response.

Norepinephrine, while sharing some functions with epinephrine, has a more targeted impact. Its primary role lies in the regulation of blood pressure and maintaining vascular tone. It powerfully constricts blood vessels throughout the body, raising blood pressure. Unlike epinephrine's focus on increased cardiac output and glucose release, norepinephrine's effects are more focused on regulating the vascular system. This is essential because maintaining blood pressure is critical for ensuring blood flow to the brain and vital organs during stressful situations. Therefore, while both catecholamines contribute to the "fight-or-flight" response, their roles differ slightly, with norepinephrine primarily managing vascular tone and blood pressure.

The precise regulation of catecholamine release is critical; excessive or insufficient levels can lead to serious health consequences. The process is complex, involving several feedback loops and neurotransmitters. The sympathetic nervous system, primarily through preganglionic cholinergic neurons, stimulates the adrenal medulla to release catecholamines. This neural control is rapid and allows for immediate responses to stressful stimuli. However, other factors, such as circulating cortisol levels, also influence catecholamine secretion. This hormonal influence contributes to a more sustained stress response and maintains the heightened state of alertness for a longer period than simply neural stimulation. Understanding these regulatory mechanisms is crucial for comprehending the body's adaptive response to stress and the potential implications of imbalances.

The adrenal medulla itself is a fascinating structure, composed primarily of chromaffin cells. These specialized cells, derived from neural crest cells, synthesize and store epinephrine and norepinephrine in secretory vesicles. Upon stimulation, these vesicles release their contents into the bloodstream, initiating the cascade of physiological effects previously described. The adrenal medulla's close anatomical relationship with the adrenal cortex highlights the intricate interplay between the glucocorticoids (cortisol) and the catecholamines. Cortisol, released from the cortex, potentiates the effects of catecholamines, contributing to the overall response to stress. The integrated response of both the adrenal cortex and medulla exemplifies the body's complex and highly organized stress response system.

In essence, the "fight-or-flight" response, mediated by the catecholamines produced by the adrenal medulla, is a finely tuned, adaptive mechanism that prepares the body for immediate action. The coordinated release of epinephrine and norepinephrine, governed by complex neural and hormonal feedback loops, ensures that the body responds effectively to a wide range of stressors, from physical threats to psychological challenges. However, chronic activation of this system, a common feature of modern life, can lead to detrimental health consequences. Understanding the physiology of the "fight-or-flight" response is crucial for appreciating the impact of stress on the human body and for developing strategies to mitigate its potentially damaging effects. The intricacy and importance of this process underscores the significance of the adrenal medulla within the broader context of adrenal function. Further exploration into the impact of chronic stress and its influence on catecholamine regulation remains an area of ongoing research, continually shaping our understanding of this crucial system. The complexity of the system requires further study, and the potential benefits for treatment and better understanding are substantial.

4.1 Epinephrine's Impact

Epinephrine, also known as adrenaline, is a crucial hormone secreted by the adrenal medulla, a vital component of the adrenal gland. Its primary role lies in mediating the body's acute stress response, often referred to as the "fight or flight" reaction. This rapid response system prepares the body for immediate action in the face of perceived danger. The surge of epinephrine triggers a cascade of physiological changes designed to enhance the body's ability to react swiftly and effectively.

This potent hormone exerts its influence through binding to specific adrenergic receptors located throughout the body. These receptors, categorized as alpha and beta receptors, are differentially distributed across various tissues and organs. This distribution accounts for the diverse physiological effects of epinephrine. For example, the activation of beta-adrenergic receptors in the heart leads to an increased heart rate and contractility, boosting cardiac output and ensuring adequate blood supply to vital organs.

Conversely, the stimulation of alpha-adrenergic receptors causes vasoconstriction in certain peripheral blood vessels, redirecting blood flow towards the heart, brain, and muscles – areas critical for immediate action. This prioritization of blood flow enhances the body's capacity to respond to the stressor effectively. Simultaneously, epinephrine impacts other physiological processes. It promotes bronchodilation, widening the airways to facilitate increased oxygen intake. This is a critical adaptation during periods of intense physical activity or respiratory distress.

Epinephrine's effects extend beyond the cardiovascular and respiratory systems. It also influences metabolic processes, mobilizing energy stores for immediate use. This mobilization involves the breakdown of glycogen into glucose in the liver, leading to an increase in blood glucose levels. This readily available glucose provides the muscles with a crucial energy source for rapid movement and sustained effort during the fight or flight response. Furthermore, epinephrine contributes to the breakdown of fats, providing an alternative energy substrate. These combined effects guarantee a sustained supply of energy to support the body's immediate needs during stress.

The regulation of epinephrine secretion is a complex interplay of neural and hormonal mechanisms. The primary regulator is the sympathetic nervous system, which responds to stressful stimuli by activating the adrenal medulla. This activation triggers the release of epinephrine into the bloodstream. Furthermore, feedback loops involving other hormones and neurotransmitters contribute to the fine-tuning of epinephrine secretion, ensuring a balanced response to various stressors. Understanding these regulatory pathways is crucial for appreciating the hormone's intricate role in maintaining homeostasis.

Beyond its acute stress response role, epinephrine plays other important functions. Its involvement in long-term adaptation to stress is becoming increasingly recognized. Chronic exposure to elevated epinephrine levels, however, can have detrimental consequences. These long-term consequences can include an increased risk of cardiovascular diseases such as hypertension and coronary artery disease. Imbalances in epinephrine levels have also been implicated in various other disorders and conditions. Therefore, maintaining appropriate epinephrine levels is crucial for overall health and well-being. In clinical settings, carefully controlled administration of epinephrine can be life-saving. It is frequently used in emergency situations, such as anaphylactic shock, to counteract life-threatening allergic reactions, for example.

The precise mechanisms through which epinephrine exerts its various effects are continuously being investigated. Detailed studies continue to elucidate the interactions between epinephrine and its receptors, providing a deeper understanding of the intricate signaling pathways involved. Moreover, researchers are actively exploring the potential therapeutic applications of epinephrine analogues and related compounds for treating a range of disorders involving cardiovascular, metabolic, and respiratory issues. A comprehensive understanding of epinephrine's impact is critical for both understanding normal physiological functioning and addressing pathological conditions.

This comprehensive insight into epinephrine's functions and impact provides a foundation for understanding how the adrenal medulla interacts with the rest of the body in maintaining homeostasis and responding to stress. Moreover, it highlights the critical need for balanced regulation of this crucial hormone to prevent the long-term health consequences associated with chronic imbalances. Future research will likely shed further light on the precise mechanisms of epinephrine action, furthering our understanding of this remarkable hormone and its vital role in human physiology. Further study into epinephrine's interactions with other hormonal systems will no doubt provide a more complete picture of its physiological role. It is an exciting field with much to uncover still.

4.2 Norepinephrine's Role

Norepinephrine, a crucial catecholamine hormone, plays a multifaceted role extending far beyond its contribution to the classic "fight-or-flight" response. While epinephrine's role is often highlighted for its widespread effects, norepinephrine exerts more localized, yet equally vital, influences on the body's physiological functions. Its actions primarily impact the nervous system, mediating both peripheral and central nervous system activities. Understanding its complexities is crucial to comprehending overall adrenal function.

Unlike epinephrine, which is predominantly released into the bloodstream for widespread effects, norepinephrine's release is more targeted. It acts as a neurotransmitter within the central nervous system, affecting mood, attention, and arousal. The precise regions influenced by norepinephrine within the brain dictate its specific impact on cognitive processes; for example, its presence in the locus coeruleus impacts vigilance and alertness. This neurotransmitter role distinguishes norepinephrine from epinephrine, contributing to its crucial role in maintaining neurological homeostasis. Moreover, its effects extend beyond the brain, influencing the autonomic nervous system and impacting cardiovascular function.

Its impact on the cardiovascular system is pronounced. Norepinephrine acts directly on the heart and blood vessels, increasing heart rate and contractility. This response results in elevated blood pressure, preparing the body for increased physical activity or stress. Simultaneously, its effects on peripheral blood vessels constrict blood flow to non-essential organs while directing more blood flow to the muscles, brain, and other vital organs, a physiological adaptation vital to meet the demands of a stressful situation. This precise vascular regulation further differentiates norepinephrine's actions from the more generalized effects of epinephrine.

Beyond its acute effects in the fight-or-flight response, norepinephrine plays a significant role in long-term physiological regulation. Its involvement in stress response pathways is intricate and prolonged. Chronic elevations in norepinephrine can have significant consequences, contributing to the development of various health issues including hypertension and cardiovascular disease. The long-term effects of sustained high norepinephrine levels underscore the importance of maintaining a balanced physiological state, emphasizing the need for stress management techniques.

Clinical implications of norepinephrine imbalances are significant. Deficiencies can lead to various neurological symptoms such as fatigue, depression, and decreased cognitive function. Conversely, excessive norepinephrine levels, frequently associated with pheochromocytoma, cause hypertensive crises with potentially life-threatening complications. Monitoring norepinephrine levels, though not as routine as cortisol or aldosterone, is crucial in diagnosing and managing specific conditions. Diagnosing conditions associated with norepinephrine imbalances requires a nuanced approach, often involving a combination of blood tests, urinary tests and careful clinical evaluations.

In summary, norepinephrine is not merely a component of the acute stress response; it's a pivotal regulator of numerous physiological processes, impacting both the nervous and cardiovascular systems. Its localized effects within the central nervous system, and its targeted actions on the periphery, highlight its essential role in maintaining homeostasis. Understanding the complexities of norepinephrine's role is crucial for appreciating the intricate workings of the adrenal medulla and its profound influence on overall health and well-being. The study of this hormone and its interactions with other systems continues to provide crucial insights into physiological mechanisms and disease processes. Further research continues to unravel more subtle and long-term effects of this fascinating hormone. The intricate pathways involved in its synthesis, release, and action provide fertile ground for future therapeutic advancements.

4.3 Stress Response

The adrenal medulla, nestled within the adrenal glands, is the powerhouse behind our immediate stress response. When faced with a perceived threat—a looming exam, a public speaking engagement, or a sudden physical danger—the sympathetic nervous system springs into action. This activation triggers a cascade of events, culminating in the release of adrenaline (epinephrine) and noradrenaline (norepinephrine) into the bloodstream. These potent catecholamines rapidly increase heart rate and blood pressure, diverting blood flow to muscles and enhancing alertness. This physiological shift prepares us for "fight or flight," an evolutionary mechanism designed to ensure survival.

These hormones don't merely act as a simple switch. Their effects are intricately woven into our body's complex network of physiological processes. Epinephrine, in particular, significantly boosts our metabolic rate, leading to increased glucose production and availability. This sudden surge of energy fuels our muscles, providing the necessary power for immediate action. The increased heart rate, propelled by both epinephrine and norepinephrine, ensures rapid oxygen delivery to working muscles. Our senses become heightened; we become more alert and focused, ready to respond to the immediate crisis.

However, the body's response to stress isn't just about physical changes. The emotional and psychological components are equally crucial. The release of catecholamines triggers the release of other hormones, like cortisol, which further amplifies the stress response. While these hormones are essential for survival in acute stressful situations, chronic stress can lead to detrimental health consequences. The persistent elevation of catecholamines places a significant burden on the cardiovascular system, increasing the risk of hypertension, heart disease, and stroke. The constant activation of the stress response suppresses the immune system, making us more vulnerable to infections and illnesses. Moreover, prolonged exposure to high levels of these hormones can negatively impact mental well-being, potentially contributing to anxiety, depression, and other mental health issues.

Understanding the intricate mechanisms of the stress response is paramount. While the "fight or flight" reaction is a powerful and often life-saving mechanism, chronic stress undermines health and well-being. It's crucial to recognize the physiological changes that accompany the stress response and to develop effective coping mechanisms. Regular exercise, proper nutrition, sufficient sleep, and stress-reducing techniques like meditation or mindfulness can help to mitigate the negative impact of chronic stress. These practices promote healthy levels of catecholamine release, enabling the body to manage stress effectively without compromising long-term health.

The body's response to stress is more nuanced than simply adrenaline. The hypothalamic-pituitary-adrenal (HPA) axis also plays a crucial role, orchestrating a slower, more sustained response. This involves the release of corticotrophin-releasing hormone (CRH) from the hypothalamus, stimulating the pituitary gland to produce adrenocorticotropic hormone (ACTH). ACTH then travels to the adrenal cortex, prompting the release of cortisol. Cortisol, unlike the rapid-acting catecholamines, has more widespread effects, influencing metabolism, immune function, and even cognitive processes.

Therefore, while catecholamines provide the immediate burst of energy for immediate action, cortisol supports a more sustained physiological response to stress. This sustained response helps to maintain energy levels, suppress inflammation, and regulate blood pressure. But, similar to catecholamines, chronically elevated cortisol levels lead to numerous adverse health effects, ranging from weight gain and insulin resistance to increased risk of cardiovascular diseases and mental health disorders. Managing stress effectively through lifestyle changes and stress reduction techniques helps regulate both catecholamine and cortisol levels, reducing the risk of these adverse consequences.

Maintaining a healthy lifestyle is vital for optimal adrenal function. A balanced diet rich in fruits, vegetables, and whole grains provides essential nutrients that support adrenal health. Regular physical activity not only helps manage stress but also strengthens the cardiovascular system, reducing its vulnerability under prolonged stress. Adequate sleep allows the body to repair and restore itself, crucial for coping with daily stressors. Incorporating relaxation techniques like meditation, deep breathing exercises, and yoga into one's routine can significantly reduce stress levels, preventing the chronic activation of the stress response. This multifaceted approach ensures that the body's inherent stress response mechanism functions optimally without overwhelming the system.

It's vital to remember that individual responses to stress vary considerably. Genetic predispositions, personal experiences, and environmental factors can all influence how our bodies respond. Some individuals might exhibit a heightened stress response, while others may appear less sensitive. Recognizing your own stress response pattern is crucial for developing personalized strategies to manage stress effectively. Seeking professional guidance, whether from a physician, therapist, or counselor, is often beneficial in developing tailored approaches to stress management and addressing any underlying mental or physical health concerns that might exacerbate the effects of stress on the adrenal system. This personalized approach can lead to improved health and well-being, enhancing the resilience of your body to daily stressors.

4.4 Adrenal Medulla

The adrenal medulla, nestled within the adrenal gland, is a vital component of the body's stress response system. Unlike the cortex, which produces steroid hormones, the medulla is primarily responsible for the synthesis, storage, and release of catecholamines: epinephrine (adrenaline) and norepinephrine (noradrenaline). These hormones are crucial for orchestrating the body's "fight-or-flight" response, a cascade of physiological changes that prepare the organism for immediate action in the face of perceived danger. This rapid response is mediated by the sympathetic nervous system, which directly innervates the chromaffin cells—specialized neuroendocrine cells—found within the medulla.

Unlike the slower-acting steroid hormones produced by the adrenal cortex, the effects of epinephrine and norepinephrine are almost immediate. Stimulation of the medulla by the sympathetic nervous system triggers the release of these hormones directly into the bloodstream. This rapid delivery allows for immediate physiological adjustments, maximizing the body's chances of survival in a threatening situation. Think of it as the body's rapid-response team, swiftly mobilizing resources to meet a perceived threat. The heart rate increases, breathing quickens, blood is shunted to the muscles, and glucose is released from the liver—all essential adaptations for immediate physical exertion.

Epinephrine, the dominant catecholamine released by the adrenal medulla, exerts a wide array of effects throughout the body. It acts primarily on alpha\item and beta-adrenergic receptors, located on the surfaces of cells in various organs. Binding to these receptors triggers intracellular signaling pathways, ultimately leading to the observed physiological changes. For instance, binding to beta-adrenergic receptors in the heart increases heart rate and contractility, while binding to beta-adrenergic receptors in the bronchi causes bronchodilation—widening of the airways, facilitating increased oxygen uptake. Meanwhile, norepinephrine, while released in smaller quantities compared to epinephrine, plays a crucial role in maintaining vascular tone, affecting blood pressure and distribution. These combined effects are critical for managing the immediate demands of the stress response.

The precise regulation of catecholamine release is essential to prevent excessive or inappropriate activation of the stress response. This intricate control is achieved through a complex interplay of neural and hormonal signals. The sympathetic nervous system, acting via preganglionic cholinergic neurons, directly stimulates the release of catecholamines from chromaffin cells. The intensity and duration of this stimulation depend on the nature and severity of the stressor, ensuring a finely tuned response to the demands of the situation. Moreover, feedback mechanisms also contribute to the regulatory process. For example, elevated levels of circulating catecholamines can negatively feedback on the sympathetic nervous system, dampening the response and preventing overstimulation.

This intricate balance ensures that the stress response is effectively controlled and avoids deleterious effects of prolonged activation.

Understanding the adrenal medulla's role in the body's stress response is crucial for comprehending various physiological and pathological conditions. Chronic or excessive activation of the sympathetic nervous system can contribute to conditions such as hypertension, anxiety disorders, and even cardiovascular disease. Conversely, impaired function of the adrenal medulla can manifest as an inability to mount an effective stress response, leaving the individual vulnerable to the detrimental effects of chronic stress. Furthermore, understanding the biochemical pathways involved in catecholamine synthesis and release is vital for the development of therapeutic interventions targeting adrenal medullary function.

Beyond the immediate "fight-or-flight" response, the adrenal medulla also plays a significant role in the body's homeostatic regulation. The continuous low-level release of catecholamines contributes to the maintenance of blood pressure, vascular tone, and metabolic processes. This subtle, yet constant, influence underlines the medulla's importance in maintaining overall physiological balance. Therefore, studying the adrenal medulla is not just about understanding stress responses, but also about grasping a core aspect of the body's overall regulatory mechanisms. Its interaction with other endocrine systems further complicates, yet enhances, the complexity of its functions within the human body. Disruption to the delicately balanced interplay of hormones within this system can lead to significant health problems.

Finally, research into the adrenal medulla continues to uncover new insights into its intricate workings and its connections to other physiological systems. Future research is likely to further illuminate the complexities of catecholamine action, revealing even more about its impact on health and disease. This ongoing exploration will undoubtedly shape future therapeutic approaches to conditions related to adrenal medullary function. The continued study of this critical organ will undoubtedly provide even deeper insights into the complexities of the human body's regulatory systems and how they relate to both health and disease. The ongoing research and understanding of the adrenal medulla's complex and vital role within the body's intricate framework continue to reveal fascinating insights that shape our approach to the treatment and management of a wide range of health conditions.

4.5 Regulation of Catecholamines

The precise regulation of catecholamine release is crucial for maintaining homeostasis and responding effectively to stress. Think of it as a finely tuned orchestra; a chaotic surge of these hormones would be disastrous, while insufficient release could leave you vulnerable. This intricate control system involves several key players, acting in concert to ensure a balanced response.

Neural control plays a pivotal role. Pre-ganglionic sympathetic neurons, originating in the spinal cord, directly innervate chromaffin cells within the adrenal medulla. The release of acetylcholine at these synapses triggers rapid catecholamine secretion, initiating the immediate "fight-or-flight" response. This is your body's immediate alarm system, preparing you for immediate action. The speed and intensity of this response are critical, highlighting the importance of immediate neural feedback loops. The brain constantly monitors internal and external cues, adjusting the signal accordingly.

However, the story doesn't end with the nervous system; endocrine mechanisms are also vital. The adrenal medulla isn't operating in isolation; it interacts dynamically with other endocrine organs. For instance, cortisol, released from the adrenal cortex, acts synergistically with catecholamines, enhancing their effects on metabolism and cardiovascular function. This collaborative effort reflects the intricate interplay of the endocrine system. Cortisol doesn't simply work independently; it modulates and amplifies the effects of other hormonal responses.

Furthermore, negative feedback loops play a critical role in preventing excessive catecholamine release. Elevated levels of circulating epinephrine and norepinephrine can trigger the release of inhibitory factors, damping down further secretion. This is a self-regulating mechanism; a brake system preventing runaway responses. These regulatory mechanisms are crucial in preventing harmful overstimulation of the heart and other organs. The body is constantly monitoring hormonal levels and acting to maintain equilibrium.

Understanding the interplay of these mechanisms is paramount for comprehending various physiological and pathological conditions. For example, during chronic stress, the sustained activation of the sympathetic nervous system can lead to dysregulation of catecholamine release, potentially contributing to hypertension, cardiovascular disease, and other health problems. In essence, the body's carefully crafted hormonal balance can be easily disrupted by long-term stress. The balance is delicate, and long-term imbalances can have far-reaching consequences.

Conversely, conditions like pheochromocytoma, characterized by an adrenal medulla tumor, result in excessive catecholamine secretion, manifesting as episodic or sustained hypertension, palpitations, and severe headaches.

The tumor disrupts the normal feedback systems, leading to uncontrolled hormone production. Therefore, understanding the fine-tuning of catecholamine regulation is essential for understanding both normal physiology and the pathogenesis of various endocrine disorders. This knowledge is crucial for diagnosis, developing effective therapeutic interventions, and, ultimately, for improving patient outcomes. The body's intricate system for regulating catecholamines underscores the importance of maintaining hormonal balance.

Beyond the immediate hormonal interactions, several other factors influence catecholamine secretion. Dietary factors, such as caffeine and certain amino acids, can indirectly affect catecholamine synthesis and release. Genetic factors also play a role, influencing the efficiency of enzymatic pathways involved in catecholamine metabolism. Moreover, environmental factors, including exposure to stress, pollutants, and sleep disruption, can profoundly impact the body's response and, subsequently, its hormone regulation. These subtle influences highlight the complexity of catecholamine regulation. Understanding these intricate interactions is paramount for developing comprehensive approaches to managing conditions related to hormone imbalances. The picture is multifaceted; multiple influences shape the body's response to internal and external stimuli.

In summary, the regulation of catecholamines is a complex, finely tuned process involving a delicate interplay of neural and endocrine mechanisms. Understanding this intricate system is pivotal for comprehending both normal physiological function and the pathogenesis of various disease states. From the immediate effects of neural stimulation to the long-term consequences of chronic stress and genetic predispositions, a holistic perspective is necessary for appreciating the intricacies of this critical endocrine system. Therefore, careful consideration of all influencing factors is crucial for both clinical practice and future research endeavors in endocrinology. The interplay of these components requires a deep understanding to effectively address health concerns arising from hormone imbalance. Continuous research and investigation are necessary to further elucidate the complexities of this system and improve treatment strategies for related disorders.

5 Adrenal Disorders

Addison's disease, a primary adrenal insufficiency, arises from the adrenal glands' inability to produce sufficient cortisol and aldosterone. This deficiency triggers a cascade of symptoms, often subtle initially, including fatigue, weakness, weight loss, and darkening of the skin. As the disease progresses, more severe manifestations appear, such as low blood pressure, salt craving, and even life-threatening adrenal crisis. Early diagnosis is crucial, utilizing blood tests to measure cortisol and ACTH levels, confirming the diagnosis and guiding treatment. This involves lifelong hormone replacement therapy, meticulously managing cortisol and aldosterone levels to mimic physiological function and prevent crises. Patient education is paramount, emphasizing prompt recognition of symptoms, emphasizing the importance of carrying a steroid emergency kit, and fostering a strong relationship with their healthcare provider.

Cushing's syndrome, on the other hand, represents the opposite spectrum – an excess of cortisol. This overproduction, stemming from various causes including adrenal tumors or prolonged corticosteroid use, leads to a characteristic set of symptoms. Weight gain, particularly around the midsection, coupled with a round face ("moon face") and fat deposits on the back of the neck ("buffalo hump"), are hallmark signs. Muscle weakness, thin skin prone to bruising, and hypertension are also frequent occurrences. Diagnosis involves a multi-faceted approach, including blood tests measuring cortisol levels and urinary cortisol excretion, alongside imaging techniques such as CT or MRI scans to identify potential tumors. Treatment strategies vary depending on the underlying cause, ranging from surgery to remove tumors to medication to suppress cortisol production or manage its effects. Close monitoring is essential, balancing the need for effective treatment with the risks of potential side effects.

Pheochromocytoma, a less common adrenal disorder, presents a unique challenge. Originating from chromaffin cells within the adrenal medulla, these tumors produce excessive catecholamines—epinephrine and norepinephrine—leading to episodic or sustained hypertension. The hallmark symptom is paroxysmal hypertension, characterized by sudden surges in blood pressure accompanied by palpitations, headache, sweating, and anxiety. Diagnosis involves careful consideration of the patient's symptoms, followed by biochemical testing, including 24-hour urine collection to measure catecholamine and metanephrine levels. Imaging studies such as CT or MRI scans are crucial to precisely locate and characterize the tumor. Surgical removal is the primary treatment, addressing the root cause of catecholamine overproduction. Preoperative management of blood pressure is paramount to minimize the risks associated with surgery and the potential for hypertensive crisis. Post-operative monitoring ensures complete tumor resection and effective control of hypertension. Understanding the unique characteristics of these three adrenal disorders—their distinct pathophysiology, clinical presentations, and diagnostic and treatment approaches—is essential for effective clinical management.

5.1 Addison's Disease

Addison's disease, also known as primary adrenal insufficiency, arises from the adrenal glands' inability to produce sufficient cortisol and aldosterone. This deficiency stems from the autoimmune destruction of adrenal cortical cells, a process where the body's own immune system mistakenly attacks these vital glands. The resulting hormone shortage profoundly impacts multiple bodily systems, causing a cascade of symptoms. Understanding the underlying pathology is crucial for effective diagnosis and management.

Unlike the other adrenal disorders, Addison's disease frequently progresses slowly and subtly, making early detection challenging. Initial symptoms often mimic other conditions, leading to delays in diagnosis. Fatigue is a common early complaint, often dismissed as stress or lifestyle factors. Weight loss, despite a normal or even increased appetite, might occur due to impaired metabolic processes. Gastrointestinal issues such as nausea, vomiting, and abdominal pain can also develop, further adding to the complexity of initial presentation. These initial signs are often nonspecific and therefore can be easily missed.

As the disease progresses, more severe symptoms appear. These include hypotension, or low blood pressure, due to the reduced aldosterone levels, impacting sodium and potassium balance. This can lead to dehydration and even circulatory collapse in severe cases. Hyperpigmentation, a darkening of the skin, especially in sun-exposed areas, is a characteristic sign often observed in Addison's disease, resulting from increased production of melanocyte-stimulating hormone (MSH). This hormone is often released in higher quantities when ACTH, the hormone responsible for stimulating cortisol production, remains chronically elevated. This highlights the intricate hormonal feedback loops involved.

The diagnostic process involves a combination of clinical evaluation, laboratory testing, and imaging studies. A thorough medical history and physical examination are essential, aiming to uncover the characteristic symptoms. Laboratory tests, like measuring cortisol and ACTH levels, are critical in confirming the diagnosis. The classic finding is low cortisol and elevated ACTH levels, indicating the adrenal glands' failure to respond appropriately to ACTH stimulation. Further testing, like the cosyntropin stimulation test, can help distinguish between primary and secondary adrenal insufficiency. Imaging studies, such as CT or MRI scans, might be used to rule out other conditions or identify adrenal gland abnormalities. A comprehensive approach ensures a precise diagnosis and guides subsequent management.

Managing Addison's disease centers on hormone replacement therapy, aiming to compensate for the deficient cortisol and aldosterone. Lifelong glucocorticoid and mineralocorticoid replacement is typically required. This usually involves taking hydrocortisone, a synthetic cortisol, and fludrocortisone, a synthetic aldosterone. Careful monitoring and dose adjustments are vital to ensure adequate hormone levels while minimizing adverse effects. Furthermore, patient education plays a crucial role, teaching individuals how to adjust medication dosages in response to illness or stress. This empowers patients to actively participate in their own care, managing their condition effectively. This active participation is crucial for successful long-term outcomes. The goal of treatment is to maintain adequate hormone levels, preventing acute adrenal crises and promoting overall well-being.

Acute adrenal crisis is a life-threatening complication of Addison's disease that requires immediate medical attention. It can be triggered by various factors such as infection, trauma, surgery, or even stress. Symptoms include severe hypotension, shock, abdominal pain, vomiting, and altered mental status. Immediate intravenous hydrocortisone administration is essential to stabilize the patient and counteract the effects of hormone deficiency. Rapid treatment is crucial for preventing fatal outcomes. Therefore, patients with Addison's disease should always carry emergency medication and seek immediate medical care at the first sign of an adrenal crisis. This awareness and preparedness are essential for long-term health and safety. Ongoing management and close monitoring are key components for a positive prognosis.

5.2 Cushing's Syndrome

Cushing's syndrome arises from prolonged exposure to high levels of cortisol, a steroid hormone primarily produced by the adrenal glands. This excess cortisol, regardless of its cause, significantly impacts nearly every system within the body, leading to a constellation of symptoms that often go unnoticed initially, hindering timely diagnosis. The insidious nature of the disease underscores the importance of recognizing its subtle yet telltale signs.

The underlying causes are diverse, ranging from benign adrenal tumors (adenomas) to cancers, and even exogenous causes like prolonged corticosteroid medication use. Understanding these different etiologies is crucial for selecting the most appropriate treatment strategy. For instance, surgically removing a benign adrenal adenoma is a definitive cure, whereas managing Cushing's syndrome induced by medication requires careful tapering of the drug dosage under close medical supervision.

Patients often present with a characteristic, moon-shaped

face, a redistribution of fat to the abdomen and the back of the neck (causing a "buffalo hump"), and thin extremities. Easy bruising and impaired wound healing are common complaints, reflecting the impact of excess cortisol on connective tissue and collagen synthesis. Furthermore, muscle weakness and osteoporosis may develop due to cortisol's catabolic effects on muscle protein and bone density. These are just a few of the possible manifestations, highlighting the systemic nature of this disorder.

The diagnostic process involves a careful evaluation of the patient's history, physical examination, and a series of laboratory tests. Blood tests are used to measure cortisol levels, both in the morning and at midnight, helping to assess the diurnal rhythm (the natural fluctuation of hormone levels throughout the day). A 24-hour urine cortisol test provides a comprehensive assessment of total cortisol production over a longer period. Imaging techniques, such as computed tomography (CT) or magnetic resonance imaging (MRI) scans, are essential for identifying adrenal tumors or other structural abnormalities in the adrenal glands.

Treatment strategies vary considerably depending on the underlying cause and the severity of the condition. For patients with adrenal adenomas, surgery is often the preferred approach, offering a potential cure by removing the source of excess cortisol. In cases where surgery is not an option, or the cause is exogenous, medical management aims to reduce cortisol levels while minimizing adverse effects. This can involve the use of medications like ketoconazole or metyrapone, which inhibit cortisol synthesis, or mifepristone, which blocks the effects of cortisol at the receptor level.

Careful monitoring is critical throughout the treatment process. Regular follow-up appointments are essential to assess the patient's response to therapy, adjust medication doses as needed, and detect any potential complications. These regular check-ups allow for early intervention should problems arise, improving overall prognosis and quality of life. The long-term management of Cushing's syndrome often requires a multidisciplinary approach involving endocrinologists, surgeons, and other specialists, ensuring that the patient receives comprehensive and tailored care.

Lifestyle modifications, including dietary changes and regular exercise, can play a supportive role in managing the condition. A healthy diet, emphasizing fruits, vegetables, and lean protein, can help to maintain a healthy weight, improve bone density, and support overall well-being. Regular exercise enhances muscle strength and improves cardiovascular fitness. However, it's crucial to remember that lifestyle changes alone are generally insufficient to control Cushing's syndrome and should always be implemented in conjunction with medical treatment, under strict medical supervision. The goal is to achieve a balance between controlling the underlying cause of the excess cortisol and managing its consequences.

The psychological impact of Cushing's syndrome should not be underestimated. The physical symptoms, along with the chronic nature of the disease and the need for ongoing medical management, can significantly affect patients' quality of life, leading to depression, anxiety, and other psychological challenges. Psychological support, in the form of counseling or therapy, can prove beneficial for patients coping with the emotional burden of this chronic disorder. Addressing these psychological aspects is just as essential as addressing the physical manifestations for complete patient well-being. It's important to remember that successful management of Cushing's syndrome is a collaborative process that requires the combined efforts of patients and their healthcare team.

5.3 Pheochromocytoma

Pheochromocytoma is a rare neuroendocrine tumor originating in the adrenal medulla, though extra-adrenal locations are possible. It's characterized by the excessive and often paroxysmal production of catecholamines, epinephrine and norepinephrine, leading to a wide array of potentially life-threatening symptoms. Understanding this condition requires a thorough grasp of both its underlying pathophysiology and its clinical manifestations.

The hallmark of pheochromocytoma is the episodic release of catecholamines, causing dramatic fluctuations in blood pressure and other physiological parameters. These "spells" can range in severity from mild headaches and palpitations to severe hypertensive crises, potentially resulting in stroke, heart failure, or even death. Between these episodes, patients may appear asymptomatic, making diagnosis challenging. The unpredictable nature of these attacks necessitates careful diagnostic evaluation and a comprehensive understanding of the condition's variability.

Diagnosis typically involves a combination of clinical suspicion and biochemical testing. A detailed patient history, focusing on symptoms such as hypertension, headaches, sweating, palpitations, and anxiety, is crucial. The classic triad of headache, sweating, and tachycardia isn't always present, highlighting the need for a high index of suspicion, especially in patients presenting with unexplained or resistant hypertension. Biochemical confirmation usually involves measuring plasma or urine catecholamines and their metabolites, such as metanephrines and vanillylmandelic acid (VMA). These measurements help quantify the extent of catecholamine overproduction.

Imaging studies play a vital role in localizing the tumor. Computed tomography (CT) scans and magnetic resonance imaging (MRI) are commonly used to visualize the adrenal glands and identify any masses. In some cases, more specialized techniques such as 123I-metaiodobenzylguanidine (MIBG) scintigraphy may be employed. This nuclear medicine procedure uses a radiotracer that targets neuroendocrine tissues, improving the detection of pheochromocytomas, especially those that are smaller or located outside the adrenal glands. Accurate localization is paramount for surgical planning, ensuring complete resection of the tumor.

Treatment for pheochromocytoma centers primarily on surgical removal of the tumor. However, pre-operative management is critical to control blood pressure and minimize the risks associated with surgery. Alpha-adrenergic blockers are typically initiated several weeks before surgery to reduce peripheral vasoconstriction and prevent hypertensive complications during the procedure. Beta-blockers are generally avoided until adequate alpha-blockade is achieved, as their use without prior alpha-blockade could worsen vasoconstriction and lead to serious cardiovascular consequences. Careful monitoring of blood pressure and other vital signs is essential throughout the pre-operative phase, adjusting medication as needed to maintain stable hemodynamic parameters.

Post-operative care involves close monitoring for recurrence and potential complications. Patients often require ongoing blood pressure management, and follow-up imaging studies are crucial to ensure complete tumor resection. Regular screening for recurrence is also recommended, given the potential for multifocality or extra-adrenal lesions in some cases. Long-term surveillance ensures early detection of any residual or recurrent disease, enabling prompt intervention and optimal patient outcomes.

The rarity of pheochromocytoma makes it a diagnostic challenge, requiring clinicians to maintain a high degree of suspicion. A comprehensive understanding of the clinical presentation, biochemical testing, and imaging techniques is crucial for timely diagnosis and appropriate management. Multidisciplinary collaboration between endocrinologists, surgeons, and anesthesiologists is essential to ensure optimal patient care, particularly during the critical perioperative phase. The ultimate goal is complete tumor resection, minimizing the risk of perioperative complications and ensuring long-term disease control. The complexities of this rare condition underscore the importance of a thorough knowledge of adrenal physiology and pathology for effective medical intervention. Successful management relies not only on technological advancements in diagnostic imaging and surgical techniques but also on a robust understanding of the pathophysiological mechanisms driving the condition. Therefore, continued research and improved clinical awareness are vital for optimizing the diagnosis, treatment, and overall outcome of patients afflicted with this potentially life-threatening disorder.

6 Adrenal Testing & Diagnosis

Accurate diagnosis of adrenal disorders relies on a combination of meticulous history-taking, physical examination, and sophisticated laboratory investigations. Blood tests form the cornerstone of adrenal testing, providing crucial insights into hormone levels and metabolic parameters. Measuring cortisol levels, both in the morning and following a stimulation or suppression test, helps differentiate between various adrenal conditions. For instance, low cortisol levels in the morning, coupled with a poor response to ACTH stimulation, strongly suggest Addison's disease. Conversely, elevated cortisol levels, often accompanied by altered glucose metabolism, may point towards Cushing's syndrome. Furthermore, precise measurements of aldosterone and renin activity are critical for assessing mineralocorticoid function and diagnosing conditions like primary hyperaldosteronism (Conn's syndrome). Analyzing the levels of dehydroepiandrosterone sulfate (DHEA-S) can contribute to evaluating adrenal androgen production.
The interpretation of these blood test results requires careful consideration of the patient's clinical presentation and other laboratory findings. Isolated abnormalities

may necessitate further investigations, including specialized tests to assess the functionality of specific enzymatic pathways within the adrenal glands. These advanced tests often involve measuring precursor and by-product hormones, providing a more granular understanding of the underlying pathophysiology. For example, assessing 17-hydroxyprogesterone levels aids in the diagnosis of congenital adrenal hyperplasia. The clinical utility of these investigations is undeniable. These tests, when correctly interpreted, offer invaluable guidance in determining the optimal treatment strategies for each patient.

Beyond blood tests, imaging techniques are indispensable in visualizing the adrenal glands and detecting structural abnormalities. Computed tomography (CT) scans provide high-resolution images, enabling the identification of adrenal adenomas, carcinomas, or hyperplasia. Magnetic resonance imaging (MRI) offers superior soft tissue contrast, particularly useful in differentiating between benign and malignant lesions. Furthermore, adrenal venous sampling, a more invasive procedure, can precisely locate the source of hormone overproduction in cases of bilateral adrenal hyperplasia or in situations where localization using imaging alone is ambiguous. This method involves the selective catheterization of the adrenal veins to measure hormone concentrations directly at the source, yielding invaluable information for surgical planning.

These imaging techniques are not used in isolation; they complement blood test findings. For example, a patient with suspected Cushing's syndrome might undergo a CT scan to visualize the adrenal glands, ruling out adrenal adenomas as the cause of elevated cortisol levels. If imaging is unrevealing, further investigations including 24-hour urine cortisol testing and a low-dose dexamethasone suppression test may be pursued. The choice of imaging modality often depends on factors such as the patient's clinical presentation, the suspected diagnosis, and the availability of resources. In some cases, a combination of CT and MRI scans might be necessary to provide a comprehensive assessment.

The integration of both blood tests and imaging techniques is crucial for a comprehensive evaluation of adrenal function. The synergy between these diagnostic tools allows clinicians to refine diagnoses, identify underlying causes of adrenal disorders, and guide the selection of appropriate treatment strategies. While blood tests offer biochemical insights into hormone levels and metabolic processes, imaging studies provide crucial structural information, enabling precise visualization of the adrenal glands and the identification of any abnormalities. This combined approach leads to a more precise diagnosis, ultimately leading to improved patient outcomes and effective management of adrenal disorders. A thorough understanding of these various diagnostic modalities is essential for any healthcare professional involved in the care of patients with suspected adrenal dysfunction. Remember, always interpret test results within the broader clinical context of the individual patient. The goal is always to provide a precise diagnosis and develop an appropriate treatment plan that optimizes the patient's health and well-being.

6.1 Blood Tests

Blood tests are invaluable tools in assessing adrenal gland function. They provide a snapshot of hormone levels, offering crucial insights into the body's hormonal balance. Understanding the specific tests and their interpretations is critical for accurate diagnosis and effective management of adrenal disorders.

A cornerstone of adrenal testing is the measurement of

cortisol levels. This is typically done via a serum cortisol test, often performed at different times of the day to account for cortisol's natural diurnal rhythm. Low cortisol levels may suggest Addison's disease, while elevated levels could indicate Cushing's syndrome. The results are interpreted considering the patient's clinical presentation and other diagnostic findings.

Beyond cortisol, measuring adrenocorticotropic hormone (ACTH) is vital. ACTH, produced by the pituitary gland, stimulates cortisol release. High ACTH levels with low cortisol suggest primary adrenal insufficiency (Addison's disease), while low ACTH levels with low cortisol indicate secondary adrenal insufficiency (a problem with the pituitary gland itself). This distinction is crucial for guiding appropriate treatment.

Aldosterone levels are assessed to evaluate mineralocorticoid function. An aldosterone test, often conducted in conjunction with a renin test, helps diagnose primary aldosteronism (Conn's syndrome), a condition characterized by excessive aldosterone production. The renin level helps differentiate between primary and secondary forms of aldosteronism. Interpretation of these results demands a deep understanding of the renin-angiotensin-aldosterone system.

Catecholamine measurements are essential for diagnosing pheochromocytoma, a rare but potentially life-threatening tumor of the adrenal medulla. This involves measuring levels of epinephrine, norepinephrine, and metanephrines (metabolic byproducts of catecholamines) in urine or plasma. Elevated levels strongly suggest a pheochromocytoma, prompting further investigation and often surgical intervention. This testing requires specialized laboratories to ensure accuracy.

Assessing 24-hour urine collection of cortisol and catecholamines provides a comprehensive evaluation of adrenal hormone production over a longer period. This method provides a more representative assessment of hormone production compared to single time point measurements, allowing for detection of subtle fluctuations that might otherwise be missed. Accurate urine collection is paramount for reliability, thus careful patient instruction is vital.

Beyond hormone levels, certain metabolic markers can provide valuable supplemental information. For example, assessing serum electrolytes like sodium, potassium, and chloride can give indirect clues about aldosterone and cortisol function. Abnormalities in these electrolytes can indicate underlying adrenal dysfunction and guide further investigation. This approach enhances the diagnostic process by integrating information from multiple parameters.

Furthermore, certain antibody tests may be necessary to distinguish between different forms of adrenal insufficiency. Antibodies against adrenal enzymes can indicate autoimmune adrenalitis, which is a major cause of Addison's disease. These additional investigations are crucial for determining the underlying cause of the adrenal dysfunction and for tailoring treatment accordingly. A thorough history and careful evaluation of symptoms are key factors to consider.

In summary, blood tests are central to the evaluation of adrenal disorders. Cortisol, ACTH, aldosterone, renin, and catecholamine levels along with urine studies and electrolyte assessments are key components of a comprehensive evaluation. Understanding the nuances of these tests, their interpretation, and their clinical correlation is crucial to the proper diagnosis and treatment of a range of adrenal conditions. Proper test selection and interpretation require a solid understanding of endocrinology and a collaborative approach involving clinicians and laboratory specialists. The complexity of these tests demands specialized training and a careful consideration of the patients individual history and symptoms. This allows healthcare professionals to utilize blood tests most effectively and tailor diagnostic strategies to individual cases, offering the highest chance of success in both diagnosis and treatment plans. The careful use of blood testing procedures is therefore paramount in the field of adrenal medicine. Remember, these are only tools and clinical judgment is also indispensable in the diagnosis process. Only through careful interpretation and integration with other aspects of patient evaluation can a complete and accurate diagnosis be achieved.

6.2 Imaging Techniques

Imaging techniques are crucial for visualizing adrenal glands and detecting abnormalities. They provide essential information supplementing blood tests, allowing for a comprehensive assessment of adrenal health. Radiographic imaging, such as X-rays, while useful in detecting calcifications, offers limited detail for adrenal gland evaluation. Computed tomography (CT) scans, however, provide excellent anatomical detail, revealing the size, shape, and internal structure of the adrenal glands. CT scans can effectively identify adrenal masses, even small ones, differentiating between adenomas, carcinomas, and other lesions. Contrast agents used with CT can further enhance visualization and improve the identification of hypervascular lesions indicative of certain adrenal tumors, particularly pheochromocytomas.

Magnetic resonance imaging (MRI) offers another powerful approach. Unlike CT scans which utilize ionizing radiation, MRI relies on magnetic fields and radio waves, making it a safer alternative, especially for patients requiring repeated scans. MRI provides superior soft-tissue contrast, allowing for better differentiation between various adrenal tissues. Specific MRI sequences can reveal detailed information about adrenal gland composition and blood flow, aiding in the characterization of different types of tumors and helping distinguish between benign and malignant lesions. Functional MRI (fMRI) might also be employed to study the dynamic activity of the adrenal glands, although this application remains more specialized.

Ultrasound, a non-invasive imaging technique, utilizes high-frequency sound waves to generate images of internal organs. It's readily available, relatively inexpensive and can be utilized as a first-line imaging modality, particularly for suspected adrenal masses that are palpable during a physical examination. Although its resolution is lower compared to CT and MRI, ultrasound can help guide needle biopsies, facilitating the histopathological examination of suspicious lesions. The procedure's non-invasive nature makes it suitable for initial assessment and follow-up evaluations.

Nuclear medicine imaging techniques, such as adrenal scintigraphy or I-131 MIBG scans, play a unique role in adrenal imaging. These techniques utilize radioactive tracers that are selectively taken up by adrenal cells, allowing for visualization of adrenal function and identification of specific types of tumors. I-131 MIBG scans, for example, are particularly useful in detecting pheochromocytomas and neuroblastomas, as these tumors avidly uptake the tracer. Adrenal scintigraphy helps identify areas of abnormal cortisol or aldosterone production, aiding in the diagnosis of specific adrenal disorders.

Choosing the most appropriate imaging technique depends on the clinical context, the specific questions being addressed, the patient's overall health, and the availability of resources. For example, if a patient presents with suspected pheochromocytoma, I-131 MIBG scintigraphy might be prioritized. If an adrenal mass is detected incidentally, a CT scan might initially be preferred for its high resolution and ability to distinguish anatomical features. The combination of various imaging modalities, along with clinical assessment and hormonal assays, often leads to the most comprehensive and accurate diagnosis. This multi-modal approach helps to minimize diagnostic uncertainty and enables the appropriate selection of therapeutic strategies. Careful integration of imaging data with clinical findings and other diagnostic tests is paramount in the diagnosis and management of adrenal disorders. The choice isn't simply about picking the best single test, but about understanding how each technique contributes to the bigger picture, ultimately leading to better patient outcomes. Therefore, a collaborative approach between radiologists, endocrinologists, and other healthcare professionals is essential to ensure optimal patient care.

7 Therapeutic Interventions

Managing adrenal disorders requires a multifaceted approach, tailored to the specific condition and the individual's needs. Medication plays a crucial role, forming the cornerstone of many treatment plans. For instance, in Addison's disease, lifelong glucocorticoid and mineralocorticoid replacement is essential, meticulously mimicking the body's natural hormone production. Careful monitoring of hormone levels is vital, ensuring the dosage remains appropriately adjusted to maintain optimal health and prevent adverse effects. Similarly, Cushing's syndrome necessitates medication to control cortisol overproduction, often involving medications that suppress adrenal hormone synthesis or block cortisol's effects. These medications require careful titration and close observation for side effects.

Lifestyle interventions are equally important, complementing medication and often significantly improving outcomes. A balanced diet, rich in fruits, vegetables, and lean protein, helps maintain healthy body weight and reduces the metabolic burden on the adrenal glands. Regular exercise, while adjusted to the individual's capabilities, strengthens the body's ability to manage stress and improves overall wellbeing. Stress management techniques, such as yoga, meditation, or mindfulness exercises, help modulate the hypothalamic-pituitary-adrenal (HPA) axis, mitigating excessive cortisol production that often exacerbates adrenal disorders. Quitting smoking and limiting alcohol consumption are further crucial lifestyle changes. These modifications contribute significantly to overall health, improving the patient's quality of life and supporting the effectiveness of any medications.

Surgical interventions are sometimes necessary, particularly in cases of adrenal tumors like pheochromocytoma or adrenal adenomas causing hormonal imbalances. Adrenalectomy, the surgical removal of one or both adrenal glands, is considered when medical management proves inadequate or in situations of malignancy. Preoperative preparation is crucial, including medication to control blood pressure fluctuations often associated with pheochromocytoma. Postoperative care includes careful monitoring of hormone levels and diligent replacement therapy to avoid adrenal insufficiency. While surgery offers definitive treatment for some conditions, it necessitates careful consideration of potential risks and benefits and should be undertaken only when medically indicated.

Hormone replacement therapy is vital in cases of adrenal insufficiency, like Addison's disease, and after adrenalectomy. This involves administering synthetic glucocorticoids and mineralocorticoids to replace the hormones the body is no longer producing adequately. The goal is to restore hormonal balance and alleviate symptoms, thereby improving the patient's overall health and well-being. Precise dosage adjustment is crucial to minimize side effects while ensuring adequate replacement. Regular blood tests are essential for monitoring hormone levels and ensuring optimal treatment efficacy, frequently adjusting doses to meet the patient's changing needs. Long-term adherence to hormone replacement therapy is necessary for maintaining health and preventing life-threatening complications.

Emerging research offers hope for future advancements in the treatment of adrenal disorders. Scientists are exploring novel therapeutic agents that target specific pathways involved in hormone regulation, potentially offering more precise and effective treatments with reduced side effects. Gene therapy holds promise for addressing genetic defects underlying some adrenal conditions. Furthermore, innovative diagnostic techniques, such as advanced imaging and molecular biomarkers, are being developed to improve early detection and personalize treatment strategies. The continual advancement of research paves the way for improved treatment outcomes and an enhanced quality of life for individuals facing adrenal disorders. These advancements are crucial for managing these complex endocrine conditions more effectively.

7.1 Medication Management

Managing adrenal disorders often requires medication, a crucial aspect of therapeutic intervention. The specific medications and dosages depend heavily on the underlying condition, the individual's unique response, and the severity of symptoms. Close monitoring by a physician is therefore essential to ensure optimal treatment and minimize potential side effects. Regular blood tests are vital to track hormone levels and adjust medication as needed.

For instance, in Addison's disease, where the adrenal glands don't produce enough cortisol and aldosterone, hormone replacement therapy is the cornerstone of treatment. This typically involves taking hydrocortisone, a synthetic cortisol, to replace the body's deficient production.

The dose is carefully adjusted based on individual needs and may vary throughout the day to mimic the body's natural cortisol rhythm. Fludrocortisone, a synthetic aldosterone, is also often prescribed to manage salt and water balance.

Cushing's syndrome, characterized by excess cortisol, presents a different challenge. Medication management focuses on reducing cortisol levels. This might involve medications like ketoconazole, an antifungal drug that can also inhibit cortisol production, or metyrapone, which blocks cortisol synthesis. Alternatively, surgery to remove a cortisol-producing tumor is often the preferred treatment, particularly when a benign adrenal adenoma is identified as the cause. Surgery is often accompanied by medication to control adrenal function until a normal state can be re-established.

Pheochromocytoma, a tumor of the adrenal medulla that produces excessive catecholamines, necessitates a different treatment strategy. Alpha-adrenergic blockers, like phenoxybenzamine, are frequently used to control high blood pressure associated with excessive catecholamines. These medications work by blocking the effects of norepinephrine and epinephrine on blood vessels, helping to lower blood pressure gradually before surgery to remove the tumor. Beta-blockers, such as propranolol, are usually added after blood pressure is controlled with alpha-blockers, to help manage the increased heart rate and other symptoms. The surgical removal of the tumor is often the definitive treatment for pheochromocytoma, once the pre-operative blood pressure has been stabilized with medications.

Beyond these specific conditions, medication management plays a role in addressing other adrenal-related issues. For example, medications targeting symptoms like high blood pressure or elevated blood sugar can be necessary.

Anti-inflammatory drugs may be indicated to manage any inflammation resulting from hormonal imbalances. Each case requires a comprehensive evaluation by an endocrinologist to determine the appropriate course of action.

It's crucial to understand that medication management is not a standalone treatment. It's typically part of a broader therapeutic strategy that may also include lifestyle adjustments and, in some cases, surgery. The success of treatment heavily relies on patient adherence to the prescribed medication regimen and regular follow-up appointments with their healthcare provider. Open communication with your physician and a thorough understanding of your medication is essential for successful management of your condition.

Effective management also involves a proactive approach to recognizing and reporting any side effects. Medications can cause various side effects, ranging from mild discomfort to more serious complications. Prompt reporting of any new or worsening symptoms is vital to allow for timely adjustment of the medication or investigation of other underlying issues. For instance, steroid medications like hydrocortisone can cause mood swings, weight changes, and increased risk of infections. Regular monitoring of these factors enables adjustments to be made before these effects become major problems.

Remember, self-medicating is extremely dangerous when dealing with hormonal imbalances. The interplay of hormones in the body is complex, and incorrect medication or dosage can lead to dangerous consequences. Always consult a physician before starting or stopping any medication, even over-the-counter remedies, to prevent unintended interactions or adverse reactions. Following your doctor's instructions meticulously is paramount to effective and safe management of any adrenal disorder.

Moreover, understanding how your medications interact

with other aspects of your life, such as diet and exercise, is crucial. This includes recognizing that certain foods, supplements, or even other medications might interfere with the effectiveness of your adrenal medication. Consulting with a registered dietitian or pharmacist can provide valuable insights into such interactions and inform healthy choices that support treatment. This holistic approach underscores the importance of a proactive and informed partnership between the patient and their healthcare team in managing adrenal conditions. Effective treatment goes beyond mere medication; it encompasses an understanding of lifestyle factors and their impact on your overall health.

Finally, remember that the road to recovery isn't always straightforward. There might be periods of adjustment, where medication dosages need to be fine-tuned to find the optimal balance. Patience and persistence, coupled with close collaboration with your healthcare team, are essential for achieving and maintaining good health. Regular monitoring of hormone levels and careful attention to any side effects are key aspects of a successful long-term treatment plan. Don't hesitate to ask questions and voice concerns. Your healthcare providers are there to support you throughout your journey.

7.2 Lifestyle Changes

Regular physical activity is crucial. Aim for at least 150 minutes of moderate-intensity aerobic exercise or 75 minutes of vigorous-intensity aerobic exercise per week, spread throughout the week. This helps regulate cortisol levels, reducing the risk of adrenal fatigue and improving overall stress management. Incorporate strength training exercises at least two days a week, targeting all major muscle groups. Building muscle mass boosts metabolism and improves insulin sensitivity, beneficial for managing blood sugar levels, often affected in adrenal disorders. Remember to consult your physician before starting any new exercise regimen, particularly if you have pre-existing health conditions. Listen to your body, and don't push yourself too hard, especially when starting. Gradual progression is key to preventing injuries and burnout.

Prioritizing sleep is paramount. Aim for 7-9 hours of quality sleep each night. Sleep deprivation significantly impacts cortisol levels, leading to increased stress and potentially exacerbating adrenal issues. Establish a regular sleep schedule, even on weekends, to regulate your body's natural circadian rhythm. Create a relaxing bedtime routine, perhaps including a warm bath, reading a book, or listening to calming music. Optimize your sleep environment; ensure your bedroom is dark, quiet, and cool. Consider using earplugs or an eye mask to block out distractions. If you struggle with insomnia or sleep disorders, consult a healthcare professional for guidance and potential treatment options, such as cognitive behavioral therapy for insomnia. Adequate sleep profoundly impacts your overall health and well-being, particularly for individuals with adrenal concerns.

Nutrition plays a vital role in adrenal health. Focus on a balanced diet rich in whole foods, including plenty of fruits, vegetables, lean proteins, and whole grains. These provide essential nutrients for adrenal function and overall well-being. Limit processed foods, refined sugars, and excessive caffeine intake, as these can negatively impact hormone balance and stress levels. Prioritize nutrient-dense foods: Include foods rich in vitamin C, B vitamins, magnesium, and zinc, as these support adrenal function. Consider incorporating foods rich in antioxidants to combat oxidative stress, which can further impact adrenal health. Regular meals and snacks throughout the day can help prevent blood sugar fluctuations, reducing stress on the adrenal glands. Consulting a registered dietitian or nutritionist can provide personalized dietary guidance tailored to your individual needs and health conditions.

Stress management is absolutely essential. Chronic stress is a major contributor to adrenal dysfunction. Implement stress-reducing techniques into your daily life, such as yoga, meditation, deep breathing exercises, or spending time in nature. Engage in activities you enjoy as a means of relaxation and stress relief. Prioritize mindfulness practices to cultivate self-awareness and improve emotional regulation. Learning to say "no" to commitments that overwhelm you is also crucial in stress management. Set realistic boundaries and learn to delegate tasks when necessary. Building strong social connections and maintaining positive relationships provides emotional support and reduces stress. Consider seeking professional help from a therapist or counselor to develop coping mechanisms for stress and improve mental well-being, especially if stress feels overwhelming or unmanageable.

Hydration is often overlooked, but crucial for optimal adrenal function. Aim to drink plenty of water throughout the day, at least eight glasses. Dehydration can exacerbate stress on the adrenal glands, leading to fatigue and other symptoms. Electrolytes, especially sodium, potassium, and magnesium, are important for adrenal function. Maintain healthy electrolyte balance through a balanced diet or, if necessary, supplementation under medical supervision. Avoid excessive alcohol consumption, as it can dehydrate the body and negatively impact adrenal function. Pay attention to your body's signals of thirst, and drink water regularly, even before feeling thirsty. Adequate hydration is vital for overall health and well-being, especially in supporting the function of your adrenal glands.

7.3 Surgical Options

Surgical intervention in adrenal disorders represents a last resort, typically reserved for cases unresponsive to medical management. The specific procedure depends heavily on the underlying condition and the extent of the adrenal gland involvement. For instance, in cases of pheochromocytoma, a tumor of the adrenal medulla secreting excess catecholamines, surgical removal—adrenalectomy—is often the primary treatment, aiming to control the often life-threatening effects of hypertension and arrhythmias. Careful preoperative preparation is vital, often involving medications to stabilize blood pressure before surgery. The success of the surgery hinges on complete tumor removal, minimizing the risk of recurrence. Post-operative monitoring is equally important, closely watching for complications such as hemorrhage or infection.

Adrenalectomy, the removal of all or part of an adrenal gland, may be necessary in cases of Cushing's syndrome where medication proves insufficient in controlling excess cortisol production. The decision involves careful weighing of the potential benefits of hormone control against the risks associated with adrenal insufficiency. This procedure may involve unilateral adrenalectomy, removing the affected gland, or bilateral adrenalectomy, a more extensive procedure requiring lifelong hormone replacement therapy. Bilateral adrenalectomy is typically reserved for severe cases with bilateral adrenal hyperplasia or when the affected glands are significantly enlarged, leading to compression of nearby structures.

A less invasive approach, particularly suitable for smaller

adrenal adenomas or tumors, is laparoscopic adrenalectomy. This minimally invasive surgery uses smaller incisions and specialized instruments, leading to reduced pain, faster recovery time, and a shorter hospital stay, when compared to open surgery. The laparoscopic approach utilizes a camera inserted through a small incision to guide the surgeon. This allows for a precise surgical removal of the affected tissue, often leaving healthy adrenal tissue untouched. However, the feasibility of a laparoscopic approach depends on factors such as tumor size and location, as well as the surgeon's experience. This method is contraindicated in certain cases.

Surgical removal may also be considered for specific adrenal masses, even in the absence of overt hormonal symptoms. This is frequently employed when imaging reveals a suspicious lesion and it proves difficult to confirm a diagnosis through non-invasive methods. Such cases necessitate careful consideration, balancing the potential risks of surgery against the small but real risk of malignant transformation. It's crucial to remember that regular follow-up imaging is critical after surgery, particularly for benign lesions or tumors, monitoring for any signs of recurrence or new growth.

Finally, one must emphasize the crucial role of preoperative hormonal evaluation and subsequent careful post-operative management. This includes detailed assessment of hormone levels to guide treatment and monitor for complications. In cases where complete adrenalectomy is performed, lifelong hormone replacement therapy is essential to ensure proper bodily function, addressing the absence of cortisol and aldosterone. The replacement therapy must carefully mimic the natural rhythm of hormone production and will require regular adjustments to ensure optimal hormone levels. Post-operative recovery, while varying between patients, involves monitoring for bleeding, infections, and ensuring patients receive suitable pain management and support as they adapt to life following this significant surgery. Careful monitoring of electrolyte balance and blood pressure is also important and must remain a priority in the post-operative phase.

7.4 Hormone Replacement

Hormone replacement therapy is a cornerstone of managing adrenal insufficiency, a condition resulting from insufficient cortisol and aldosterone production. Successfully implementing this therapy necessitates a thorough understanding of the individual's specific needs, carefully monitored dosage adjustments, and vigilant observation for adverse effects. The goal is to mimic the body's natural hormone production as closely as possible, restoring homeostasis and improving quality of life. This requires a tailored approach rather than a one-size-fits-all solution.

The most common form involves replacing both cortisol and aldosterone. Hydrocortisone, a synthetic cortisol analogue, is typically administered orally, often in divided doses to better mirror the body's natural diurnal rhythm. The dosage must be carefully titrated, starting low and gradually increasing based on clinical response and laboratory monitoring. This is essential to avoid both under-replacement, which leaves symptoms unresolved, and over-replacement, which can lead to serious side effects. Regular blood tests, measuring cortisol levels and electrolytes, are vital to fine-tune the dose and ensure efficacy.

Aldosterone replacement is usually necessary only in cases of significant mineralocorticoid deficiency. Fludrocortisone acetate is the most commonly used medication, a potent synthetic mineralocorticoid, helping restore sodium and potassium balance. Its administration requires careful monitoring of blood pressure and electrolytes, with potassium levels carefully watched for hyperkalemia, a dangerous elevation of potassium. Similar to hydrocortisone, dosage adjustments are incremental, guided by the patient's response and laboratory data. The process is not simply a matter of prescribing a medication; rather it requires a constant monitoring of the body's response and a flexible approach.

Beyond medication, patient education is crucial. Understanding the importance of adhering to the prescribed regimen is paramount. Patients need clear instructions on medication administration, potential side effects (such as weight gain, mood changes, or fluid retention), and the importance of consistent follow-up appointments for monitoring. Open communication with the healthcare provider to address any concerns or challenges is indispensable in long-term adherence.

Lifestyle adjustments also play a role in managing adrenal insufficiency. Maintaining a balanced diet is beneficial, providing the body with the nutrients necessary for optimal function and potentially helping minimize some medication side effects. Stress management techniques, including yoga, meditation, or mindfulness practices, can also be helpful, as stress can exacerbate adrenal insufficiency symptoms. Regular exercise, within one's capabilities, promotes overall well-being and can contribute to better health outcomes. This comprehensive approach, encompassing medication, monitoring, and lifestyle modification, represents the best practice in adrenal insufficiency management.

Patients with Addison's disease, a primary form of adrenal insufficiency, require lifelong hormone replacement. The precise dosage varies greatly depending on individual factors, including age, weight, overall health, and the severity of the disease. Careful monitoring is vital because even minor fluctuations in dosage can lead to significant changes in the individual's health.

During times of illness or increased stress, patients often require supplemental doses of hydrocortisone to counteract the increased demand on the adrenal glands. This "stress dosing" can be crucial during periods of increased stress or illness to prevent adrenal crisis, a life-threatening condition characterized by dangerously low cortisol levels. Patients should be carefully educated about the need for stress doses and how to adjust their medication appropriately, especially during times of illness or major stress. They must understand their personal stress dose requirements and carry emergency medication when traveling or engaging in potentially stressful activities.

Furthermore, regular follow-up appointments with an endocrinologist are essential for continued monitoring of hormone levels, blood pressure, and overall health. These appointments allow for ongoing adjustments to medication, addressing any potential complications, and ensuring that the therapy remains effective and safe over the long term. Close collaboration between patient and healthcare provider remains a central element in long-term success with hormone replacement therapy. This approach, which embraces personalized treatment and comprehensive monitoring, ensures patients receive the support they need to live full and productive lives. It is not just a medical intervention, but a collaborative effort aimed at empowering individuals to manage their condition effectively.

7.5 Future Treatments

Gene therapy holds immense promise. Researchers are actively exploring the use of gene therapy to correct genetic defects underlying certain adrenal disorders. This approach could potentially offer a long-term, possibly even curative, solution for conditions like congenital adrenal hyperplasia, where enzymatic deficiencies disrupt hormone production. Imagine a future where a single treatment could permanently restore normal hormone levels, eliminating the need for lifelong medication and significantly improving patient quality of life. The challenge lies in delivering the therapeutic genes effectively to the adrenal cells and ensuring long-term expression without adverse effects. However, preliminary results are encouraging, suggesting this avenue warrants further investigation. Precise gene editing techniques, like CRISPR-Cas9, are also being explored to correct specific genetic mutations, offering a more targeted approach than traditional gene therapy methods. This targeted approach could minimize potential off-target effects.

3D bioprinting is revolutionizing regenerative medicine, and its potential applications in adrenal disorders are exciting. Scientists are experimenting with bioprinting functional adrenal tissues using patient-specific cells. This would enable the creation of personalized implants to replace damaged or diseased adrenal glands. This innovative technology could overcome the limitations of current transplantation methods, reducing the risk of rejection and offering a more readily available source of adrenal tissue. Challenges remain in mimicking the complex three-dimensional structure and vascularization of the adrenal gland, which are crucial for proper hormone secretion. Further research is needed to optimize bioprinting parameters and ensure the long-term viability and functionality of the bioprinted tissues. But the potential to offer a functional replacement for damaged adrenal glands is very significant.

Stem cell therapy offers a versatile approach. Researchers are investigating the ability of different stem cell types, including induced pluripotent stem cells (iPSCs) and mesenchymal stem cells (MSCs), to differentiate into adrenal cortical cells. This means that stem cells could potentially be used to generate new adrenal cells in the laboratory, which could then be transplanted to repair damaged adrenal tissue or to supplement deficient hormone production. The advantage of this is that stem cells can be readily obtained from patients, reducing the risk of rejection. The significant hurdle is the efficient differentiation of stem cells into functional adrenal cells that produce the correct hormones in sufficient quantities. This requires significant research in order to fully understand the complex regulatory pathways involved.

Immunomodulatory therapies are a less invasive approach to treatment. Autoimmune adrenalitis, an autoimmune condition damaging adrenal glands, is a growing concern. Immunosuppressive drugs currently offer treatments that aim to lessen the damage to the adrenal glands. However, research is focused on developing more targeted immunomodulatory therapies that could specifically suppress the autoimmune response while minimizing adverse effects. This could include designing drugs that target specific immune cells or molecules involved in adrenal damage. This research is also studying the potential of using immunotherapy to prevent the initial onset of adrenal diseases by actively training the body's immune system to tolerate the adrenal gland.

Nanotechnology is shaping many fields of medicine, and adrenal research is no exception. Nanocarriers can deliver drugs or hormones directly to the adrenal glands, improving treatment efficacy and reducing side effects. These microscopic carriers can be designed to target specific adrenal cells and protect the drug from degradation. Nanotechnology could also facilitate the development of nanosensors that monitor hormone levels in real-time, enabling personalized treatment adjustments. The challenges involve overcoming the obstacles to safely deliver nanoparticles to the adrenal glands, and ensuring the long-term stability of the nano-based treatment. However, the potential for effective, localized therapies is substantial.

The integration of artificial intelligence and machine learning in adrenal research is offering substantial advantages. AI algorithms are being used to analyze large datasets of patient information, identifying patterns and biomarkers that could predict adrenal disease risk or treatment response. This will lead to more accurate diagnoses and personalized treatment plans based on each patient's unique characteristics. These advances will lead to a better understanding of the complex interplay of genetics, environment, and lifestyle factors that contribute to adrenal disorders. This allows for the creation of individualized preventative strategies and treatments. Furthermore, AI can accelerate drug discovery by identifying potential drug candidates and predicting their efficacy and safety.

The future of adrenal treatment is promising. Research into gene therapy, 3D bioprinting, stem cells, immunomodulation, and nanotechnology is unveiling novel therapeutic approaches for adrenal disorders. Combining these innovative technologies with the power of artificial intelligence offers a brighter future for individuals facing adrenal challenges. Each therapeutic approach presents its own unique set of challenges, but the potential benefits for patients are immense. Continued investment in research and development is vital to bring these promising treatments to clinical practice, improving the lives of countless individuals affected by adrenal insufficiency or other adrenal disorders. The collaborative efforts of scientists, clinicians, and technology developers will pave the way for new treatments that go beyond current therapeutic interventions and help to achieve a better quality of life for people living with adrenal conditions.

www.ingramcontent.com/pod-product-compliance
Lightning Source LLC
LaVergne TN
LVHW022020200926
848481LV00007B/2457
* 9 7 9 8 3 4 9 2 4 2 9 2 2 *